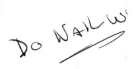

MW01226673

STATE EXAM REVIEW
FOR
NAIL TECHNOLOGY

Compiled by Barbara Jewett

Milady Publishing
(a division of Delmar Publishers)
3 Columbia Circle, Box 15015
Albany, New York 12212-5015

NOTICE TO THE READER

Publisher does not warrant or guarantee any of the products described herein or perform any independent analysis in connection with any of the product information contained herein. Publisher does not assume, and expressly disclaims, any obligation to obtain and include information other than that provided to it by the manufacturer. The reader is expressly warned to consider and adopt all safety precautions that might be indicated by the activities herein and to avoid all potential hazards. By following the instructions contained herein, the reader willingly assumes all risks in connection with such instructions.

The Publisher makes no representation or warranties of any kind, including but not limited to, the warranties of fitness for particular purpose or merchantability, nor are any such representations implied with respect to the material set forth herein, and the publisher takes no responsibility with respect to such material. The publisher shall not be liable for any special, consequential, or exemplary damages resulting, in whole or part, from the readers' use of, or reliance upon, this material.

Contents

Foreword

This book of exam reviews contains questions similar to those that may be found on state licensing exams for nail technology. It employs the multiple-choice type question, which has been widely adopted and approved by the majority of state licensing boards.

Groups of questions have been arranged under major subject areas. To get the maximum advantage when using this book, it is advisable that the review of subject matter take place shortly after its classroom presentation.

This review book reflects advances in professional nail technology. It attempts to keep pace with, and insure a basic understanding of, sanitation, anatomy, physiology and salon business applicable to the nail technician, client consultation guidelines, chemical safety in the nail salon, and basic manicuring and pedicuring procedures as well as some of the more advanced and creative aspects of the profession.

The book serves as an excellent guide for the student as well as for the experienced nail technician. It provides a reliable standard against which professionals can measure their knowledge, understanding, and abilities.

Furthermore, these reviews will help students and professionals alike to gain a more thorough understanding of the full scope of their work as they review practical performance skills and related theory. They will increase their ability to evaluate new products and procedures and to be better qualified professionals for dealing with the needs of their clients.

Chapter 1

Directions: Carefully read each statement. Insert on the blank line after each statement the letter representing the word or phrase that correctly completes the statement.

YOUR PROFESSIONAL IMAGE

1. The way you behave toward others when working in a salon is called:
   a) good will
   b) professional ethics
   c) salon conduct
   d) behavior
   _B_

2. If you keep to your appointment schedule, clients will think you are:
   a) fast
   b) competent
   c) unusual
   d) lazy
   _B_

3. The time to set up your station and sanitize your instruments is when clients are:
   a) getting coffee
   b) not yet present
   c) waiting
   d) in the bathroom
   _B_

4. Your daily schedule should include clients' names so that you can:
   a) greet them by name
   b) plan your tips
   c) get larger commissions
   d) arrange for parking
   _A_

5. When your appointments are running very late, your arriving clients should:
   a) reschedule
   b) expect shortcuts
   c) be informed
   d) go home
   _C_

6. Your attitude toward clients should always be:
   a) friendly
   b) crisp & businesslike
   c) arrogant
   d) gossipy
   _A_

7. To make them feel welcome, new clients should be:
   a) greeted by name
   b) given salon tour
   c) escorted to station
   d) all the above
   _D_

8. Mrs. Smith is always hard to please; today, she's especially difficult. In dealing with her, you should:
   a) act professionally
   b) ask her to leave
   c) yell
   d) charge her more
   _A_

9. When you are around nail chemicals, it is dangerous to:
   a) eat
   b) chew gum
   c) talk loudly
   d) smoke
   ____

10. When you communicate with your employer, no matter what the subject, you should always be:
    a) grateful for job
    b) honest
    c) assertive
    d) asking for raise
    ____

11. Your employer notices a technique you use that was developed and taught to you by a coworker. In this situation, you should tell your employer:
    a) it's your technique
    b) coworker developed technique
    c) you learned at school
    d) nothing—keep quiet
    ____

12. To get along with coworkers, you should:
   a) respect their opinions   c) buy their lunch
   b) use deodorant   d) point out mistakes
   ____

13. If you have a problem or question about your job, you should
    discuss it with:
   a) your butcher   c) your employer
   b) best friend   d) your mother   ____

14. Personal problems should always be:
   a) shared with coworkers   c) left at home
   b) shared with clients   d) told to the boss   ____

15. Learning about other services offered at the salon, such as hair and
    skin care, and then telling your clients about them, is called salon:
   a) performance   c) networking
   b) show-off   d) promotion   ____

16. Your sense of right and wrong when you interact with clients,
    employer and coworkers is called:
   a) honesty   c) moral values
   b) professional ethics   d) moodiness   ____

17. Your best source of advertising to get new clients is:
   a) radio   c) newspapers
   b) current satisfied clients   d) coupon mailers   ____

18. High ethical standards towards clients (giving them only the
    services they need and/or want) will earn you:
   a) larger commissions   c) good reputation
   b) boss's approval   d) big tips   ____

19. You have a client who is always willing to try anything you
    suggest. At her next appointment, you should give her:
   a) only needed services   c) a discount
   b) every expensive service   d) free polish   ____

20. Your state has new regulations for sanitation and safety. You
    feel many of these are unnecessary as well as inconvenient, so you:
   a) comply, it's law   c) follow some
   b) ignore them   d) quit manicuring   ____

21. Some clients love to share with you stories about your coworkers,
    your employer, or others in your community. When these clients
    start to gossip, you should:
   a) join in   c) leave station
   b) close your eyes   d) remain businesslike ____

22. For tips on keeping hands beautiful between manicures, clients
    will ask the advice of:
   a) the nail technician   c) a neighbor
   b) a coworker   d) a doctor   ____

23. You must learn the differences between salon and drugstore products in order to convince clients:
    a) to purchase higher priced products
    b) to get the best deal on products
    c) that professional products are best for nail health and beauty
    d) that drugstore products lack quality ____

24. When you and your coworkers practice professional ethics, your salon will become:
    a) well-known
    b) successful
    c) more profitable
    d) busier ____

25. Professional ethics includes keeping your:
    a) records accurately
    b) tips secret
    c) promises
    d) breaks frequent ____

26. If a client complains to you about another technician, you should:
    a) get defensive
    b) suggest client and technician talk
    c) tell your opinion
    d) call the boss immediately ____

27. You should be a model of good grooming because you are a:
    a) professional worker
    b) member of beauty industry
    c) pleasant person
    d) model ____

28. For the best professional appearance, you should be clean and fresh by bathing or showering and using a deodorant:
    a) daily
    b) once a week
    c) morning and night
    d) twice a month ____

29. The clothes you wear for work should be:
    a) very dressy
    b) spot resistant
    c) trendy
    d) clean and pressed ____

30. Female nail technicians should wear makeup to work:
    a) for special occasions
    b) once a month
    c) every day
    d) heavily applied ____

Chapter 2

BACTERIA AND OTHER INFECTIOUS AGENTS

1. One-celled microorganisms that are so small they can only be seen through a microscope are called:
   a) bugs　　　　　　　　　c) fungi
   b) parasites　　　　　　　d) bacteria　　　　D

2. Because bacteria are so small, to cover the head of a pin you would need this many of them:
   a) 2　　　　　　　　　　c) 5 million
   b) 1,500　　　　　　　　d) 10 million　　　B

3. Bacteria multiply rapidly. A single bacterial cell can produce 16 million more in only:
   a) two weeks　　　　　　c) half a day
   b) three minutes　　　　d) five days　　　　C

4. Some nonpathogenic bacteria help in:
   a) improving the fertility of soil　c) breaking down food in digestion
   b) producing food and oxygen　　d) a, b & c　　　D

5. Nonpathogenic bacteria make up nearly all bacteria, about this amount:
   a) 60%　　　　　　　　c) 50%
   b) 70%　　　　　　　　d) 100%　　　　B

6. Pathogenic bacteria are also called:
   a) microorganisms　　　c) germs
   b) cells　　　　　　　　d) toxins　　　　C

7. Disease-causing bacteria are called:
   a) bad　　　　　　　　c) secretions
   b) gross　　　　　　　d) pathogens　　　D

8. Round, pus-producing bacteria are called:
   a) cocci　　　　　　　c) influenza
   b) circular　　　　　　d) mites　　　　A

9. Baccilli are the most common bacteria, producing diseases such as tetanus, tuberculosis and:
   a) backache　　　　　　c) influenza
   b) measles　　　　　　d) cold sores　　　C

10. The common name for the disease caused by treponema pallida is:
    a) toothache　　　　　c) strep throat
    b) syphilis　　　　　　d) palsy　　　　B

11. A mature bacterial cell divides into two identical cells; this division is called:
    a) mitosis　　　　　　c) diplococci
    b) cilia　　　　　　　d) spirilla　　　　A

12. Two types of bacteria which propel themselves are bacilli and:
    a) diplococci
    b) staphylococci
    c) cocci
    d) spirilla

    _D_

13. Disease-causing agents smaller than bacteria are:
    a) viruses
    b) microbes
    c) miniatures
    d) germs

    _A_

14. Viruses enter healthy cells and:
    a) die
    b) remain the same size
    c) reproduce
    d) leave without damaging the cell

    _C_

15. The disease AIDS is caused by a:
    a) spirilla
    b) virus
    c) saprophyte
    d) spore

    _B_

16. The transfer of the HIV virus is through:
    a) sneezing
    b) common cold
    c) touching
    d) bodily fluids

    _D_

17. Nail fungus usually appears as a discoloration on the nail that spreads toward the:
    a) cuticle
    b) tip
    c) nail bed
    d) center

    _A_

18. Early stage bacterial infection can be identified as a spot which is colored:
    a) black
    b) blue
    c) yellow-green
    d) purple

    _C_

19. Clients with fungus or bacterial infection should be treated by a:
    a) manicurist
    b) optometrist
    c) cosmetologist
    d) physician

    _D_

20. The removal of artificial nails from a client with nail fungus or bacterial infection should be accomplished wearing:
    a) gown
    b) gloves
    c) mask
    d) goggles

    _B_

21. The ability of the body to resist disease is called:
    a) rickettsia
    b) infection
    c) organisms
    d) immunity

    _D_

22. After the body fights off a disease, the bloodstream contains:
    a) antibodies
    b) germs
    c) pathogens
    d) viruses

    _A_

23. Vaccines are given to artificially produce:
    a) disease
    b) fever
    c) immunity
    d) allergies

    _C_

24. Bacteria and germs multiply rapidly on:
    a) nail files
    b) cuticle nippers
    c) towels
    d) a, b & c

    _d_

25. The transfer of infected fluids between technician and client is accomplished through:
    a) drinking glasses
    b) open wounds
    c) coughing
    d) brushes

    _b_

26. The nail technician with a contagious common illness should:
    a) stay home
    b) work quickly
    c) drink juice
    d) take naps

    _d_

27. It is easy to wound a client by filing too deeply or when:
    a) removing polish
    b) massaging toes
    c) nipping cuticles
    d) applying tips

    _c_

28. Clients who fear being infected need to be:
    a) referred to a physician
    b) reassured about safety precautions
    c) distracted
    d) given health magazines to read

    _b_

29. Clients are interested in knowing:
    a) where disinfectants are stored
    b) who cleans the salon
    c) how they are at risk
    d) how you prevent the spread of disease in the salon

    _d_

30. To create a feeling of security in clients, give them specific examples of:
    a) disinfectants used
    b) disinfection procedures
    c) diseases that can be prevented
    d) treatments for nail problems

    _b_

chapter 3

SANITATION AND DISINFECTION

1. Sanitation rules are legislated and enforced for:
a) health and safety reasons   c) statistics
b) lower insurance rates   d) keeping busy   ____

2. To destroy all bacteria and make something germ-free is to:
a) sanitize   c) deodorize
b) clean   d) sterilize   ____

3. To clean and prevent germs from growing is to:
a) sterilize   c) wash
b) sanitize   d) bleach   ____

4. Antiseptics help prevent:
a) spread of viruses   c) skin infections
b) soft nail tips   d) cracked nails   ____

5. Disinfection does not kill:
a) germs   c) antibodies
b) bacterial spores   d) fungus   ____

6. A disinfectant should not come into contact with:
a) implements   c) cabinets
b) table tops   d) skin   ____

7. The Material Safety Data Sheet provides all the following EXCEPT:
a) directions for proper use   c) pricing information
b) a list of active ingredients   d) safety precautions   ____

8. Implements will contaminate disinfecting solution if they are:
a) oily   c) warm
b) wet   d) dry   ____

9. A glass receptacle which holds disinfectant and a sub-merged implement is called a/an:
a) glass   c) disinfection container
b) agent   d) antiseptic   ____

10. Cloudy solution in a disinfection container indicates:
a) contamination   c) strong solution
b) weak solution   d) ammonia   ____

11. Implements should be fully immersed in disinfecting solution for:
a) three minutes   c) ten minutes
b) six minutes   d) twelve minutes   ____

12. The most commonly used disinfectant in salons is:
a) formaldehyde   c) quats
b) bleach   d) phenolics   ____

13. The most expensive disinfectants are:
    a) alcohol and bleach
    b) phenolics
    c) antibacterial soaps
    d) quats
    ____

14. Alcohol loses effectiveness as a disinfectant when diluted below:
    a) 62%
    b) 70%
    c) 75%
    d) 85%
    ____

15. After disinfecting counter tops, you should:
    a) let them air dry
    b) leave the room for three minutes
    c) wipe with a clean towel
    d) sponge away excess disinfectant
    ____

16. When using a spray bottle for disinfectants, you should wear:
    a) gloves
    b) safety glasses
    c) an apron
    d) a mask
    ____

17. Before touching sanitized implements, the nail technician's hands should be cleaned with:
    a) ammonia
    b) bleach
    c) antibacterial soap
    d) formalin
    ____

18. Disposable items are to be discarded after use:
    a) on two clients
    b) on one client.
    c) on five clients
    d) at end of day
    ____

19. Following disinfection, dry implements should be placed in a/an:
    a) jar
    b) pocket
    c) airtight container
    d) paper towel
    ____

20. Bead "sterilizers" should not be used because:
    a) they are ineffective
    b) they are a waste of money
    c) they pose health risks
    d) a, b & c
    ____

21. Formaldehyde is a/an:
    a) safe disinfectant
    b) commonly used fumigant
    c) recommended disinfectant in all states
    d) allergic sensitizer
    ____

22. To prevent release of fumes from products used in artificial nail applications, upon completion:
    a) light a candle
    b) run air conditioner
    c) discard trash bag
    d) spray air freshener
    ____

23. Tuberculocidal disinfectants are recommended for cleaning:
    a) rest rooms
    b) blood spills
    c) doorknobs
    d) counter tops
    ____

24. If you accidentally cut a client with a file, you should:
    a) break the file and throw it away
    b) give the client the file
    c) put disinfectant on the cut
    d) disinfect the file
    ____

25. When mixing or using salon products, you should:
    a) wear gloves and safety glasses
    b) measure everything carefully
    c) read and follow instructions exactly
    d) a, b & c
    ____

26. Pouring disinfectant on your hands can:
    a) decrease the chance of infection
    b) protect your skin from pathogens
    c) cause skin disease
    d) promote good health
    ____

27. Store professional products:
    a) in a cool, dark, dry location   c) in a well-lit closet
    b) on low shelves within easy reach   d) under the sink   ____

28. Universal Sanitation includes all of the following EXCEPT:
    a) wearing gloves   c) taking short cuts
    b) using disinfectants   d) sanitizing the salon   ____

29. All of the following affect nail health EXCEPT:
    a) pregnancy   c) diet
    b) weight   d) prescription drug use   ____

30. You can custom-tailor a manicure to solve an individual's
    problems if you are:
    a) knowledgeable about nail health   c) consulting with a doctor
    b) fashion-conscious   d) using an airbrush   ____

SAFETY IN THE SALON

Chapter 4

1. Lightheadedness, runny nose, and tingling toes are symptoms of chemical:
a) burn
b) inhalation
c) overexposure
d) exposure ____

2. A Material Safety Data Sheet will tell you about a product's potential:
a) price increase
b) hazards
c) reformulation
d) discontinuation ____

3. An MSDS must include information about all of these areas EXCEPT:
a) first aid procedures
b) physical hazards
c) protection measures
d) application methods ____

4. Carcinogens are substances that can cause:
a) skin irritation
b) cancer
c) flash fires
d) spoilage ____

5. An MSDS can be obtained from your salon's:
a) distributor
b) main office
c) cleaning person
d) fire department ____

6. Nail product chemicals enter your body in all these ways EXCEPT:
a) inhalation
b) ingestion
c) injection
d) skin contact ____

7. Proper ventilation requires that fumes and vapors be vented to:
a) reception area
b) bathroom
c) outside
d) haircolor area ____

8. To be effective, the charcoal filter in a vented manicuring table must be changed every:
a) week
b) 20 hours
c) 48 hours
d) month ____

9. The area the size of a beach ball that is directly in front of your mouth is:
a) your allergy zone
b) your breathing zone
c) your health zone
d) your ventilation zone ____

10. You can eliminate vapors by all methods EXCEPT:
a) tightly sealing product containers
b) avoiding use of pressurized sprays
c) running fans
d) emptying waste containers ____

11. The best solution to salon vapor and dust control is:
a) fans
b) vented manicure table
c) local exhaust
d) blowers ____

12. The distance between a roof exhaust pipe and an intake vent should be at least:
a) eight feet
b) ten feet
c) fifteen feet
d) twenty-one feet ____

13. An accidental splash of disinfectant solution or primer can seriously injure the:
    a) nail
    b) polish
    c) implements
    d) eyes
    _____

14. To protect lungs when filing nails, you and your client should wear:
    a) dust masks
    b) bandanas
    c) oxygen tanks
    d) clean towels
    _____

15. Dust masks quickly lose effectiveness and should be replaced:
    a) every few days
    b) daily
    c) monthly
    d) yearly
    _____

16. When the possibility for chemical splashing exists, you and your client should wear:
    a) masks
    b) gloves
    c) rubber aprons
    d) eye protection
    _____

17. Because of the possibility of eye injury, contact lenses should not be worn when:
    a) skiing
    b) swimming
    c) working in the salon
    d) showering
    _____

18. Many nail products are highly flammable, thus smoking near them could cause a:
    a) ventilation overload
    b) fire
    c) skin allergy
    d) chronic cough
    _____

19. To avoid ingesting chemicals at your station, you and your clients should not:
    a) smoke
    b) breathe
    c) touch
    d) eat or drink
    _____

20. Food and chemicals in the salon should be stored in:
    a) the refrigerator
    b) paper bags
    c) separate areas
    d) the office
    _____

21. To help prevent chemical ingestion, never eat anything in the salon without first:
    a) washing hands
    b) asking permission
    c) having an antacid
    d) taking a sample
    _____

22. To prevent chemical accidents, never use a product if its container is not:
    a) sealed
    b) sanitized
    c) full
    d) labeled
    _____

23. Storage for chemicals should be in cool areas and away from:
    a) appliance/furnace with pilot light
    b) hair colors
    c) perm solutions
    d) garbage cans
    _____

24. Nail products can be ruined by:
    a) overmixing
    b) excessive heat
    c) shaking too hard
    d) cool temperatures
    _____

25. Many nail products are even more flammable than:
    a) lighter fluid
    b) charcoal
    c) water
    d) gasoline
    _____

26. To help keep your area well ventilated, empty your plastic trash bag:
    a) daily
    b) weekly
    c) several times per day
    d) monthly   ____

27. Capping products will reduce vapors and make them:
    a) look neater
    b) last longer
    c) harder to open
    d) easier to steal   ____

28. To cover the small dishes you use for acrylic powder and liquid, use:
    a) jar lids
    b) marbles
    c) plastic wrap
    d) aluminum foil   ____

29. Cumulative trauma disorders can be caused by all factors EXCEPT:
    a) chemical overexposure
    b) repetitive motion
    c) awkward twisting
    d) working in one position   ____

30. To turn safety into a promotion for nail art, add your hand-painted designs to frames of:
    a) safety goggles
    b) nail dryers
    c) dust masks
    d) chairs   ____

Chapter 5

NAIL PRODUCT CHEMISTRY SIMPLIFIED

1. Sulfur cross-links create strong:
   a) natural nails
   b) toxins
   c) odors
   d) vitamins
   ___

2. Energy has no:
   a) velocity
   b) heat
   c) substance
   d) power
   ___

3. A water molecule can be broken down into:
   a) helium and oxygen
   b) hydrogen and oxygen
   c) hydrogen and ozone
   d) helium and ozone
   ___

4. When water becomes ice, there is a:
   a) chemical change
   b) physical improvement
   c) chemical reaction
   d) physical change
   ___

5. A catalyst can make a chemical reaction:
   a) cleaner
   b) faster
   c) hotter
   d) slower
   ___

6. A substance that dissolves something is called a/an:
   a) solute
   b) enhancement
   c) catalyst
   d) solvent
   ___

7. When removing artificial nail enhancements, warming the solvent to 105° speeds removal time by:
   a) 15%
   b) 25%
   c) 30%
   d) 50%
   ___

8. A chemical that causes two surfaces to stick together is a/an:
   a) contaminant
   b) adhesive
   c) saturated solvent
   d) surfactant
   ___

9. Substances that improve adhesion are:
   a) primers
   b) solutes
   c) enhancements
   d) corrosives
   ___

10. Washing hands and scrubbing the nail plate removes:
    a) bacteria and fungal spores
    b) surface oils
    c) contaminants
    d) a, b & c
    ___

11. Adhesion is best when the nail plate is:
    a) roughed up
    b) thin
    c) cold
    d) clean and dry
    ___

12. Overfiling promotes all of the following problems EXCEPT:
    a) allergic reactions
    b) bruising
    c) infections
    d) loss of the nail plate
    ___

13. Gigantic chains of molecules are called:
    a) corrosives
    b) monomers
    c) polymers
    d) histamines
    ___

14. When an initiator touches a monomer it:
    a) destroys it
    b) energizes it
    c) tranquilizes it
    d) disables it

15. A billion monomers can join in less than:
    a) a second
    b) five minutes
    c) thirty minutes
    d) one hour

16. A monomer that joins different polymer chains is called a:
    a) bridge
    b) rung
    c) cross-linker
    d) tie

17. Light-cured enhancements generally use:
    a) sunlight
    b) ultraviolet light
    c) fluorescent light
    d) incandescent light

18. All of the following are evaporation coatings EXCEPT:
    a) nail polishes
    b) gels
    c) top coats
    d) base coats

19. The most common skin disease for nail technicians is:
    a) acne
    b) eczema
    c) psoriasis
    d) contact dermatitis

20. Sensitive clients generally show allergic symptoms after repeated exposure for:
    a) one to two months
    b) four to six months
    c) eight to nine months
    d) ten to twelve months

21. You must always leave a margin between the skin and the product of:
    a) 1/16"
    b) 1/8"
    c) 3/16"
    d) 3/8"

22. UV bulbs used to cure enhancements should be cleaned daily and changed at least:
    a) twice a month
    b) every month
    c) every three months
    d) twice a year

23. Allergic reactions are caused by all the following EXCEPT:
    a) overexposure
    b) improper product consistency
    c) any contact with monomers
    d) custom blending your own mixture

24. The number of nail technicians affected by skin disorders on their hands is:
    a) 35%
    b) 40%
    c) 50%
    d) 65%

25. When the skin is damaged by irritants, the immune system releases:
    a) histamines
    b) antibodies
    c) antitoxins
    d) hormones

26. A common salon irritant is:
    a) skin cream
    b) cuticle oil
    c) tap water
    d) rubbing alcohol

27. Prolonged or repeated contact with solvents will leave the skin:
    a) burned
    b) oily
    c) shiny
    d) dry and damaged ____

28. Product dusts and residues can accumulate on:
    a) brush handles
    b) containers
    c) table tops
    d) a, b & c ____

29. In order to sell a product you should do all of the following EXCEPT:
    a) show the client where all the products are displayed
    b) use the product in the service
    c) place the item in the client's hand
    d) ask if you can add it to the ticket ____

30. The best time to attempt to sell the product is:
    a) during the initial consultation
    b) while you use the product
    c) at the end of the manicure
    d) when you schedule another appointment ____

ANATOMY AND PHYSIOLOGY

1. The study of the structure of the body and what it is made of is called:
   a) physiology
   b) anatomy
   c) medicine
   d) physical ____

2. The study of the small, individual structures of the body, such as hair, nails, sweat glands and oil glands, is called:
   a) psychology
   b) anatomy
   c) histology
   d) microbes ____

3. An understanding of body structure will make you more proficient when doing:
   a) hand & arm massage
   b) basic manicures
   c) pedicures
   d) acrylics ____

4. The basic unit of all living things is the:
   a) tissue
   b) protein
   c) nucleus
   d) cell ____

5. The protoplasm of the cell consists of all the following EXCEPT:
   a) nucleus
   b) scilli
   c) cytoplasm
   d) centrosome ____

6. The cell is surrounded by the:
   a) nucleus
   b) protoplasm
   c) centrosome
   d) cell membrane ____

7. Cells reproduce themselves through a process called:
   a) anabolism
   b) centrosome
   c) mitosis
   d) nucleus ____

8. The chemical process whereby the body cells are nourished is called:
   a) metabolism
   b) anabolism
   c) mitosis
   d) centrosome ____

9. The maintenance of normal, internal stability in the body is called:
   a) mitosis
   b) anabolism
   c) homeostasis
   d) catabolism ____

10. The protective covering on body surfaces such as skin and mucous membranes is called:
    a) muscular tissue
    b) epithelial tissue
    c) nerve tissue
    d) connective tissue ____

11. Cartilage and ligaments are examples of:
    a) liquid tissue
    b) muscular tissue
    c) fat tissue
    d) connective tissue ____

12. Messages are carried to and from the brain by:
    a) brain tissue
    b) nerve tissue
    c) liquid tissue
    d) epithelial tissue ____

13. Structures designed to accomplish a specific bodily function are called:
    a) cells
    b) building blocks
    c) organs
    d) nuclei
    _____

14. The number of systems in the body is:
    a) 10
    b) 5
    c) 15
    d) 25
    _____

15. All of the following are bodily systems EXCEPT:
    a) integumentary
    b) circulatory
    c) synovial
    d) excretory
    _____

16. The physical foundation of the body is the:
    a) cell
    b) skeleton
    c) heart
    d) muscles
    _____

17. Bones are connected by movable and immovable:
    a) bands
    b) tissues
    c) nerves
    d) joints
    _____

18. The skeleton is composed of:
    a) 206 bones
    b) 260 bones
    c) 50 bones
    d) 157 bones
    _____

19. The only bones in the body that are not extremely hard are the:
    a) ankles
    b) teeth
    c) knees
    d) elbows
    _____

20. Bone is white on the outside; the inside is:
    a) pink
    b) blue
    c) off-white
    d) deep red
    _____

21. The pink fibrous membrane that covers and protects bone is the:
    a) periosteum
    b) cartilage
    c) muscle
    d) tendon
    _____

22. The bands of fibrous tissue which support the bones at the joints are called:
    a) cartilage
    b) ulna
    c) ligaments
    d) periosteum
    _____

23. The ankle and wrist are:
    a) pivot joints
    b) gliding joints
    c) hinge joints
    d) ball-and-socket joints
    _____

24. The large bone on the small-finger side of the forearm is the:
    a) clavicle
    b) ulna
    c) radius
    d) humerus
    _____

25. The long, slender bones of the palm and hand are:
    a) carpus
    b) phalanges
    c) metacarpals
    d) fibula
    _____

26. The common name for calcaneous is:
    a) heel
    b) cartilage
    c) elbow
    d) calf muscle
    _____

27. The long, slender bones of the foot are:
    a) metacarpals
    b) femur
    c) carpus
    d) metatarsals
    _____

28. The muscles in the human body number more than:
    a) 100
    b) 500
    c) 800
    d) 1,000 ____

29. Muscles of the face, arm and leg are:
    a) myology
    b) cardiac
    c) non-striated
    d) striated ____

30. Smooth muscles function automatically and are classified as:
    a) striated
    b) non-striated
    c) cardiac
    d) slick ____

31. Muscle tissue can be stimulated by all of the following EXCEPT:
    a) massage
    b) light rays
    c) nerve impulses
    d) phalanges ____

32. The muscle which turns the hand outward so the palm faces down is the:
    a) pronator
    b) supinator
    c) flexor
    d) extensor ____

33. The muscle which turns the hand inward so the palm faces upward is the:
    a) pronator
    b) supinator
    c) flexor
    d) extensor ____

34. The muscles which separate the fingers are called the:
    a) adductors
    b) abductors
    c) opponent
    d) flexor ____

35. The muscles which draw the fingers together are the:
    a) adductors
    b) abductors
    c) pronator
    d) flexor ____

36. The muscle attached at the rear of the heel which pulls the foot down is the:
    a) gastrocnemius
    b) soleus
    c) gluteous maximus
    d) peroneus longus ____

37. The muscle which covers the front of the shin and bends the foot upward and inward is the:
    a) soleus
    b) peroneus brevis
    c) tibialis anterior
    d) peroneous longus ____

38. The following are nervous system divisions EXCEPT:
    a) automatic
    b) cerebro-spinal
    c) neurology
    d) peripheral ____

39. Body movements are controlled by;
    a) central nervous system
    b) peripheral system
    c) sympathetic system
    d) parasympathetic system ____

40. The sympathetic division of the automatic nervous system is activated during times of:
    a) rest
    b) homeostasis
    c) stress
    d) deep thought ____

41. Nerves which carry impulses from the brain to the muscles are called:
    a) afferent nerves
    b) efferent nerves
    c) receptors
    d) mixed nerves ____

42. The nerve which supplies the fingers is the:
    a) ulnar
    b) radial
    c) digital
    d) sural   ____

43. The nerve which supplies impulses to the top of the foot is the:
    a) sural
    b) dorsal
    c) tibial
    d) saphenous   ____

44. The heart, arteries, veins, capillaries, lymph glands and lymph vessels make up the body's:
    a) circulatory system
    b) endocrine system
    c) respiratory system
    d) digestive system   ____

45. The bodily fluid which aids in protecting the body from harmful bacteria and infection through its white cells is:
    a) lymph
    b) urine
    c) water
    d) blood   ____

Chapter 7

THE NAIL AND ITS DISORDERS

1. The medical specialty that focuses on skin problems is called:
   a) urology
   b) dermatology
   c) cardiology
   d) pediatrics   ____

2. Healthy nails look:
   a) smooth, shiny and pink
   b) smooth, shiny and dull red
   c) smooth, dull and pink
   d) smooth, dull and white   ____

3. The technical term for nail is:
   a) keratin
   b) pearl
   c) onyx
   d) lunula   ____

4. Nails grow more quickly during this season:
   a) autumn
   b) winter
   c) spring
   d) summer   ____

5. The main part of the nail that is attached to the skin at the tip of the finger is the:
   a) nail root
   b) nail bed
   c) free edge
   d) nail body   ____

6. Nail growth begins at the:
   a) free edge
   b) root
   c) plate
   d) nail bed   ____

7. The end of the nail that extends beyond the fingertip is called the:
   a) matrix
   b) fold
   c) root
   d) free edge   ____

8. The portion of the skin beneath the nail body upon which rests the nail plate is called the:
   a) nail root
   b) nail bed
   c) matrix
   d) lunula   ____

9. Nail cells are produced in the nail:
   a) root
   b) matrix
   c) bed
   d) fold   ____

10. The half-moon shape at the base of the nail is called the:
    a) mantle
    b) matrix
    c) root
    d) lunula   ____

11. The loose, pliable, overlapping skin around the nail is called the:
    a) mantle
    b) matrix
    c) cuticle
    d) nail grooves   ____

12. The deep fold of skin at the base of the nail where the nail root is embedded is the:
    a) mantle
    b) matrix
    c) eponychium
    d) perionychium

13. Slits or tracks in the nail bed at the side of the nail are the:
    a) cuticle
    b) mantle
    c) nail wall
    d) nail grooves ____

14. The skin on the sides of the nail above the grooves is called:
    a) hyponychium
    b) nail wall
    c) mantle
    d) cuticle ____

15. The thin line of skin at the base of the nail that extends from the nail wall to the nail plate is the:
    a) hyponychium
    b) cuticle
    c) lunula
    d) eponychium ____

16. The part of the skin that surrounds the entire nail area is the:
    a) perionychium
    b) hyponychium
    c) eponychium
    d) nail wall ____

17. The part of the skin under the nail's free edge is called:
    a) eponychium
    b) matrix
    c) hyponychium
    d) paronychium ____

18. A nail condition caused by injury or disease is called a nail:
    a) imperfection
    b) disfigurement
    c) disorder
    d) fungus ____

19. It is safe to work on a nail with this condition:
    a) inflammation
    b) small furrows
    c) infection
    d) swelling ____

20. Inflamed skin is:
    a) infected
    b) black and blue
    c) red and sore
    d) yellow ____

21. A skin or nail infection will show evidence of:
    a) bruising
    b) pus
    c) furrows
    d) discoloration ____

22. The condition in which a clot of blood forms under the nail plate due to injury to the nail bed is called:
    a) discolored nails
    b) inflammation
    c) infection
    d) bruised nails ____

23. Nails which are thin, white and curved over the free edge are called:
    a) healthy
    b) eggshell
    c) furrowed
    d) hangnails ____

24. Hangnails are caused by:
    a) dry cuticles
    b) nail biting
    c) polish
    d) buffing ____

25. The wasting away of the nail is called:
    a) onychauxis
    b) onychatrophia
    c) onychophagy
    d) onychocryptosis ____

26. The overgrowth of nails is:
    a) onychauxis
    b) onychatrophia
    c) onychocryptosis
    d) onychophagy ____

27. Nail disorders that you cannot treat and must refer client to a doctor include all of the following EXCEPT:
    a) mold
    b) tinea unguium
    c) onychophagy
    d) pyogenic granuloma ____

28. A condition which can occur on the nails of the hands or feet is:
    a) paronychia
    b) onycholysis
    c) onychia
    d) onychoptosis _____

29. Paronychia around the entire nail is sometimes called:
    a) total infection
    b) paronychia totalis
    c) runaround
    d) onychoptosis _____

30. Onychia and paronychia are often caused by:
    a) fever
    b) infection
    c) unsanitary implements
    d) bruising _____

chapter 8

THE SKIN AND ITS DISORDERS

1. The ability of healthy skin to regain its shape immediately after being pulled away from the bone is called:
a) electricity
c) stimuli
b) elasticity
d) fluidity ____

2. The skin performs all of these jobs for the body EXCEPT:
a) protection
c) nutrition
b) heat regulation
d) excretion ____

3. The outer layer of skin is called the:
a) dermis
c) papilla
b) epidermis
d) subcutaneous tissue ____

4. The deep layer of skin is called the:
a) dermis
c) papilla
b) epidermis
d) subcutaneous tissue ____

5. The epidermis contains no:
a) nerves
c) blood vessels
b) keratin
d) cells ____

6. The waterproof coating for the skin is found in the layer of the epidermis called the:
a) stratum lucidum
c) melanin
b) stratum mucosum
d) stratum corneum ____

7. The small epidermal layer composed of clear cells is the:
a) stratum corneum
c) stratum mucosum
b) stratum lucidum
d) melanin ____

8. Cells that look like granules are in the layer of epidermis called:
a) stratum lucidum
c) stratum granulosum
b) stratum corneum
d) stratum mucosum ____

9. Melanin is found in this epidermis layer:
a) stratum lucidum
c) stratum corneum
b) stratum germinativum
d) stratum granulosum ____

10. Blood vessels and nerves are found in the:
a) dermis
c) follicle
b) epidermis
d) stratum corneum ____

11. The dermal layer which lies directly under the epidermis is the:
a) adipose tissue
c) tactile corpuscles
b) papillary layer
d) horny layer ____

12. Fat cells, blood vessels and sweat glands are found in the:
a) subcutaneous layer
c) epidermis
b) papillae
d) reticular layer ____

13. The fatty tissue found in the subcutaneous layer of the dermis is called:
    a) energy cells
    b) cellulite
    c) adipose
    d) papal ____

14. Arrector pili muscles can cause:
    a) spasms
    b) arthritis
    c) hair growth
    d) goose bumps ____

15. Sensory nerve endings are most abundant in the:
    a) toes
    b) fingertips
    c) nose
    d) eyes ____

16. The common name for the sudoriferous glands is:
    a) oil glands
    b) hormones
    c) sweat glands
    d) lymph nodes ____

17. The small opening in the skin surface through which the sudoriferous glands eliminate waste is the:
    a) papal
    b) sweat pore
    c) hair shaft
    d) secretory nerve ____

18. A structural change in tissue caused by injury and disease is called:
    a) lesion
    b) pustule
    c) fissure
    d) scar ____

19. A semi-solid or fluid lump above and below the skin surface is called a:
    a) papule
    b) macule
    c) cyst
    d) nodule ____

20. A lump on the skin with an inflamed base and a head containing pus is called a:
    a) tubercle
    b) pustule
    c) scale
    d) scar ____

21. Severe dandruff is an example of:
    a) scales
    b) crust
    c) fissure
    d) bulla ____

22. The common name for tinea pedis is:
    a) eczema
    b) athlete's foot
    c) pimple
    d) cold sore ____

23. Ringworm of the hand is highly contagious and caused by a:
    a) pigment
    b) mold
    c) scratch
    d) fungus ____

24. The congenital absence of melanin pigment in the body is called:
    a) psoriasis
    b) herpes simplex
    c) albinism
    d) vesicle ____

25. The proper name for liver spots is:
    a) chloasma
    b) vitiligo
    c) sarcoma
    d) birthmark ____

26. Darkening of the skin caused by exposure to the ultraviolet rays of the sun is called a:
    a) mole
    b) keratoma
    c) tan
    d) birthmark ____

27. People with vitiligo must be protected from:
    a) chemicals
    b) sun
    c) water
    d) freckles   ____

28. The common name for keratoma is:
    a) carotene
    b) freckles
    c) callus
    d) mol   ____

29. A round, thickened patch of epidermis due to pressure or friction in which the thickening grows inward is called a:
    a) sarcoma
    b) corn
    c) hive
    d) mole   ____

30. A fatal skin cancer which begins with the growth of a mole is called:
    a) vitiligo
    b) chloasma
    c) melanin
    d) melanotic sarcoma   ____

Chapter 9

CLIENT CONSULTATION

1. The conversation you have with a client before starting the service is called the client:
a) chat   c) service record
b) consultation   d) conduct   ____

2. During a consultation, you will need to assess all of these aspects EXCEPT:
a) client's health   c) client's lifestyle
b) client's skin   d) client's hairstyle ____

3. The difference between "doing nails" and being a professional nail technician is a good client:
a) attitude   c) consultation
b) base   d) location   ____

4. If the client has a skin or nail inflammation, you should tactfully suggest the client:
a) wash better   c) eat less salt
b) see a physician   d) stop biting nails ____

5. Performing a service on an infected nail could cause your client a great amount of:
a) happiness   c) filing
b) soaking   d) pain   ____

6. For your client's safety, always try to use products which are:
a) hypoallergenic   c) weak strength
b) new   d) lifestyle   ____

7. Before performing a nail service, make sure the home maintenance suits the client's:
a) budget   c) looks
b) wardrobe   d) lifestyle   ____

8. To determine the client's needs, you need to ask about all the following EXCEPT:
a) job   c) hobbies
b) insurance   d) household chores ____

9. If your client is a gardener, the best nail length is:
a) medium   c) short
b) long   d) nail tips   ____

10. As a professional nail technician, it is your job to make your clients:
a) happy   c) short
b) buy retail products   d) get silk wraps   ____

11. The best time to explain a service is:
a) as you perform it   c) upon completion
b) don't need to explain   d) before you start ____

12. If the client leaves the salon happy with the service, chances are good the client will:
    a) tip well
    b) return again
    c) complain
    d) bite her nails
    ____

13. Because customer loyalty is crucial to your success, you must show clients you appreciate their:
    a) promptness
    b) repeat business
    c) tips
    d) courtesy
    ____

14. You can express your appreciation to clients by:
    a) sending birthday cards
    b) sending newsletters
    c) hosting a thank-you party
    d) a, b & c
    ____

15. Client health/record cards should be kept in a location that is:
    a) convenient
    b) locked
    c) fireproof
    d) secret
    ____

16. To protect hands and nails when doing housework, clients should wear:
    a) hand lotion
    b) top coat
    c) rubber gloves
    d) clear polish
    ____

17. Client health/record cards provide the technician all the following EXCEPT:
    a) general information
    b) credit history
    c) medical information
    d) lifestyle information
    ____

18. The client's name and address are examples of:
    a) health information
    b) medical information
    c) personal data
    d) general information
    ____

19. Questions about hobbies are part of the:
    a) general information
    b) client profile
    c) medical information
    d) friendship process
    ____

20. Knowing a client's general health will indicate the safety of giving a client a:
    a) manicure
    b) pedicure
    c) hand or foot massage
    d) cuticle remover
    ____

21. Client service records are usually kept on:
    a) index cards
    b) pink paper
    c) computer
    d) duplicate forms
    ____

22. Retail products purchased should be part of the client's:
    a) consultation card
    b) receipt
    c) charge slip
    d) service record
    ____

23. When a client's regular technician is not available, the client can best be serviced by referring to the:
    a) client's hairstylist
    b) salon next door
    c) owner's instructions
    d) client's service record
    ____

24. The client health/record and the client service record should be used as:
    a) consultation tools
    b) retail boosters
    c) public information
    d) computer data base
    ____

25. Caring about the health, safety and quality of service your clients receive makes you a:
    a) slow worker
    b) professional
    c) good insurance risk
    d) supervisor
    ____

MANICURING

chapter 10

1. The number of types of nail technology tools is:
   a) three
   b) four
   c) five
   d) six

   B

2. Permanent items used in nail technology are called:
   a) implements
   b) overhead
   c) equipment
   d) materials

   C

3. The lamp on a manicure table should have a bulb with a wattage of:
   a) 40
   b) 50
   c) 60
   d) 100

   A

4. A low wattage bulb is not able to:
   a) produce sufficient light
   b) dry polish
   c) warm client's nails
   d) kill germs

   C

5. A high wattage bulb will interfere with product when performing:
   a) sculptured nails
   b) pedicures
   c) wet sanitizing
   d) polish change

   A

6. A fingerbowl is used to soak the client's fingers in warm water and:
   a) germicide
   b) dish detergent
   c) alcohol
   d) antibacterial soap

   D

7. A client cushion can be fashioned by the technician from a:
   a) pillow
   b) towel
   c) foam square
   d) cotton coil

   B

8. Implements include all the following EXCEPT:
   a) electric nail dryer
   b) orangewood stick
   c) steel pusher
   d) metal nail file

   A

9. Emery boards, orangewood sticks and cotton are items that are:
   a) reusable
   b) sterile
   c) disposable
   d) expensive

   C

10. The common name for steel pusher is:
    a) cuticle nipper
    b) cuticle pusher
    c) orangewood stick
    d) emery board

    D

11. To shape the free edge of hard or sculptured nails, use a/an:
    a) metal nail file
    b) emery board
    c) orangewood stick
    d) cuticle nipper

    A

12. A good choice for filing soft or fragile nails is a/an:
    a) metal nail file
    b) chamois buffer
    c) fingernail clippers
    d) emery board

    D

13. To lift small bits of cuticle from the nail, use a/an:
    a) cuticle nipper
    b) tweezer
    c) orangewood stick
    d) cotton ball

    B

14. It is not a good idea to save an emery board in a plastic bag for each client, due to the growth of:
    - a) papules
    - b) fungus
    - c) bacteria
    - d) parasites

    C

15. To add shine to the nail and smooth out wavy ridges, you should use a:
    - a) metal nail file
    - b) emery board
    - c) nail brush
    - d) chamois buffer

    D

16. To cut filing time on long nails, shorten nails with a:
    - a) cuticle nipper
    - b) fingernail clipper
    - c) nail buffer
    - d) metal nail file

    B

17. Materials are single-use supplies that are used during a manicure and include all the following EXCEPT:
    - a) cotton balls
    - b) towels
    - c) plastic bags
    - d) nail brush

    D

18. During a manicure, antibacterial soap is mixed with warm water and used:
    - a) sparingly
    - b) in the fingerbowl
    - c) after polish application
    - d) after top coating

    B

19. Nail cosmetics include all of the following EXCEPT:
    - a) top coat
    - b) in the fingerbowl
    - c) alcohol
    - d) cuticle oil

    C

20. The basic nail shapes include all of the following EXCEPT:
    - a) square
    - b) hexagon
    - c) round
    - d) oval

    B

21. The best nail shape for clients who work on typewriters, computers and assembly lines is:
    - a) square
    - b) round
    - c) oval
    - d) pointed

    A

22. The most common nail shape for male clients is:
    - a) square
    - b) round
    - c) oval
    - d) pointed

    B

23. The best nail shape choice for businesswomen is often:
    - a) square
    - b) round
    - c) oval
    - d) pointed

    C

24. As a professional nail technician, all services you perform will have three parts:
    - a) pre-service, manicure, post-service
    - b) consultation, procedure, retail sale
    - c) pre-service, pedicure, retail sale
    - d) pre-service, procedure, post-service

    D

25. To reduce heat during buffing, spray client's nails with:
    - a) hairspray
    - b) water
    - c) alcohol
    - d) oil

    B

26. To mix polish, you should:
    - a) shake bottle
    - b) tap bottle on table
    - c) stir with brush
    - d) roll bottle between palms

    D

27. When the entire nail plate is polished, the application is called:
    a) slimline
    b) lunula
    c) full coverage
    d) hairline tip

    C

28. The French Manicure is a great base for:
    a) pale polish
    b) buffing
    c) nail art
    d) artificial tips

    C

29. Clients with ridged and brittle nails or dry cuticles should benefit from:
    a) reconditioning hot oil manicure
    b) French Manicure
    c) gentle scrubbing
    d) gel nails

    A

30. Most men generally need more work don on their:
    a) free edge
    b) hangnails
    c) buffing
    d) cuticles

    D

31. Paraffin treatments are ideal for the:
    a) hands and feet
    b) arms and legs
    c) neck
    d) face

    A

32. Massage service stimulates:
    a) nail growth
    b) blood flow/circulation
    c) skin growth
    d) heartbeat

    B

33. The massage service should not be performed on a client with any of the following conditions EXCEPT:
    a) high blood pressure
    b) cough
    c) stroke
    d) heart condition

    B

34. Vigorous massage of joints can be painful for clients with:
    a) hangnails
    b) osteoporosis
    c) arthritis
    d) lung condition

    C

PEDICURING

chapter 11

1. Trimming, shaping and polishing toenails as well as performing foot massage is called:
   a) manicuring
   b) toe trimming
   c) podiatry
   d) pedicuring   D

2. When taking an appointment for a pedicure, tell the client polish will not smear if they:
   a) wear open-toed shoes/sandals
   b) wear cotton socks
   c) wear black hose
   d) wear pumps   A

3. The pedicuring station includes all the following EXCEPT:
   a) client chair
   b) telephone
   c) client footrest
   d) technician's chair   B

4. A properly set up pedicure station will have this many rinse and soap baths:
   a) one
   b) two
   c) three
   d) four   B

5. To remove dry skin or callus growths, use a/an:
   a) foot file
   b) antibacterial soap
   c) antiseptic spray
   d) antifungal agent   A

6. An antiseptic spray for pedicuring contains a/an:
   a) talcum powder
   b) antifungal agent
   c) antibacterial soap
   d) foot lotion   B

7. During the pedicure procedure, the client's feet should be placed on a:
   a) toe separator
   b) dry floor
   c) clean terry towel
   d) pedicure slipper   C

8. You may not perform a pedicure on a client with any of the following conditions EXCEPT:
   a) athlete's foot
   b) fungus
   c) infection
   d) hang nail   D

9. When water is spilled during pedicuring, wipe it up immediately to prevent:
   a) falls
   b) bacteria growth
   c) fungus growth
   d) athlete's foot   A

10. The purpose of soaking the feet prior to the pedicure procedure is:
    a) to remove calluses
    b) sanitation
    c) to soften hangnails
    d) to relax client   B

11. Toe separators should be inserted before this pedicure step:
    a) clipping nails
    b) removing polish
    c) brushing nails
    d) filing nails   D

12. Toenails should be filed straight across, with corners:
    a) straight
    b) square
    c) slightly rounded
    d) filed into   C

13. Cuticle solvent may be used to soften excess skin below
the nail's:
   a) free edge
   b) bed
   c) polish
   d) root

14. Most pedicure services are performed by starting with:
   a) left foot, little toe
   b) right foot, little toe
   c) left foot, big toe
   d) right foot, big toe

15. To avoid tickling client's foot during massage, use a:
   a) massage machine
   b) greasy lotion
   c) firm touch
   d) light touch

16. To avoid smearing polish, the top coat should be followed by:
   a) a second top coat
   b) instant nail dry
   c) warm blowing air
   d) cool blowing air

17. In winter, feet can suffer from:
   a) dryness
   b) cramping
   c) cracking
   d) a, b & c

18. To maintain the pedicure at home, the client should purchase
all the following products EXCEPT:
   a) polish
   b) antibacterial soap
   c) lotion
   d) top coat

19. Following a pedicure service, basins, tables and footrests should
be sanitized with:
   a) steam
   b) dry heat
   c) a hospital-grade disinfectant
   d) fungicide

20. Pedicure implements must have proper sanitation before use for
at least:
   a) 5 minutes
   b) 20 minutes
   c) 30 minutes
   d) 60 minutes

21. Between each service, your table should be arranged for:
   a) basic set-up
   b) best appearance
   c) proper sanitation
   d) clean top

22. The client with high blood pressure, heart condition or stroke
should not have a massage without permission from a:
   a) chiropractor
   b) spouse
   c) salon owner
   d) physician

23. The foot massage begins with:
   a) joint relaxer movements
   b) effleurage on top
   c) effleurage on heel
   d) metatarsal scissors

24. Clients will find effleurage:
   a) painful to joints
   b) stimulating
   c) relaxing
   d) causes burning sensation

25. To perform joint movement for toes, toes are moved so as to
create a:
   a) popping sound
   b) figure eight
   c) complete circle
   d) square

ANSWERS TO
STATE EXAM REVIEW
FOR
NAIL TECHNOLOGY

ANSWERS TO STATE EXAM REVIEW FOR NAIL TECHNOLOGY

YOUR PROFESSIONAL IMAGE

1-c	6-a	11-b	16-b	21-d	26-b	29-d
2-b	7-d	12-a	17-b	22-a	27-b	30-c
3-b	8-a	13-c	18-c	23-c	28-a	
4-a	9-d	14-c	19-a	24-b		
5-c	10-b	15-d	20-a	25-c		

BACTERIA AND OTHER INFECTIOUS AGENTS

1-d	6-c	11-a	16-d	21-d	26-a	29-d
2-b	7-d	12-d	17-a	22-a	27-c	30-b
3-c	8-a	13-a	18-c	23-c	28-b	
4-d	9-c	14-c	19-d	24-d		
5-b	10-b	15-b	20-b	25-b		

SANITATION AND DISINFECTION

1-a	6-d	11-c	16-d	21-d	26-c	29-b
2-d	7-c	12-c	17-c	22-c	27-a	30-a
3-b	8-a	13-b	18-b	23-b	28-c	
4-c	9-c	14-b	19-c	24-b		
5-b	10-a	15-a	20-d	25-d		

SAFETY IN THE SALON

1-c	6-c	11-c	16-d	21-a	26-c	29-a
2-b	7-c	12-c	17-c	22-d	27-b	30-a
3-d	8-b	13-d	18-b	23-a	28-b	
4-b	9-b	14-a	19-d	24-b		
5-a	10-c	15-a	20-c	25-d		

NAIL PRODUCT CHEMISTRY SIMPLIFIED

1-a	6-d	11-d	16-c	21-b	26-c	29-a
2-c	7-c	12-b	17-b	22-d	27-d	30-c
3-b	8-b	13-c	18-b	23-c	28-d	
4-d	9-a	14-b	19-d	24-b		
5-b	10-d	15-a	20-b	25-a		

ANATOMY AND PHYSIOLOGY

1-b	8-a	15-c	22-c	29-d	35-a	41-b
2-c	9-c	16-b	23-b	30-b	36-a	42-c
3-a	10-b	17-d	24-b	31-d	37-c	43-b
4-d	11-d	18-a	25-c	32-a	38-c	44-a
5-b	12-b	19-b	26-a	33-b	39-a	45-d
6-d	13-c	20-d	27-d	34-b	40-c	
7-c	14-a	21-a	28-b			

THE NAIL AND ITS DISORDERS

1-b	6-b	11-c	16-a	21-b	26-a	29-c
2-a	7-d	12-a	17-c	22-d	27-c	30-c
3-c	8-b	13-d	18-c	23-b	28-b	
4-d	9-b	14-b	19-b	24-a		
5-d	10-d	15-d	20-c	25-b		

THE SKIN AND ITS DISORDERS

1-b	6-d	11-b	16-c	21-a	26-c	29-b
2-c	7-b	12-d	17-b	22-b	27-b	30-d
3-b	8-c	13-c	18-a	23-d	28-c	
4-a	9-b	14-d	19-c	24-c		
5-c	10-a	15-b	20-b	25-a		

Client Consultation

1-b	5-d	9-c	13-b	17-b	21-a	24-a
2-d	6-a	10-a	14-d	18-d	22-d	25-b
3-c	7-d	11-d	15-a	19-b	23-d	
4-b	8-b	12-b	16-c	20-c		

Manicuring

1-b	6-d	11-a	16-b	21-a	26-d	31-a
2-c	7-b	12-d	17-d	22-b	27-c	32-b
3-a	8-a	13-b	18-b	23-c	28-c	33-b
4-c	9-c	14-c	19-c	24-d	29-a	34-c
5-a	10-b	15-d	20-b	25-b	30-d	

Pedicuring

1-d	6-b	11-d	16-b	21-a	26-d	29-b
2-a	7-c	12-c	17-d	22-d	27-a	30-d
3-b	8-d	13-a	18-b	23-a	28-c	
4-b	9-a	14-a	19-c	24-c		
5-a	10-b	15-c	20-b	25-b		

Nail Tips

1-b	6-c	11-b	16-b	21-d	26-d	29-d
2-c	7-b	12-c	17-b	22-a	27-c	30-a
3-b	8-a	13-d	18-b	23-b	28-b	
4-a	9-b	14-a	19-a	24-a		
5-d	10-d	15-c	20-c	25-c		

Nail Wraps

1-b	6-c	11-a	16-c	21-b	26-c	29-c
2-c	7-a	12-d	17-b	22-d	27-a	30-d
3-a	8-c	13-c	18-a	23-c	28-b	
4-d	9-b	14-b	19-d	24-b		
5-b	10-d	15-a	20-a	25-a		

ACRYLIC NAILS

1-b	6-c	11-c	16-a	21-d	26-b	31-a
2-a	7-b	12-a	17-d	22-b	27-a	32-b
3-c	8-c	13-c	18-b	23-c	28-c	
4-d	9-d	14-d	19-a	24-a	29-b	
5-a	10-a	15-b	20-c	25-d	30-d	

GELS

1-b	4-c	7-d	10-c	12-a	14-b
2-a	5-b	8-c	11-b	13-d	15-c
3-d	6-a	9-a			

THE CREATIVE TOUCH

1-a	4-b	7-c	10-a	13-a	16-a
2-b	5-d	8-b	11-c	14-b	17-a
3-c	6-a	9-d	12-b	15-c	

SALON BUSINESS

1-c	6-c	11-a	16-b	21-a	26-a	29-b
2-a	7-b	12-d	17-a	22-d	27-d	30-c
3-d	8-a	13-b	18-d	23-a	28-b	
4-a	9-d	14-a	19-b	24-c		
5-b	10-c	15-c	20-c	25-b		

SELLING NAIL PRODUCTS AND SERVICES

1-c	5-c	9-a	13-a	17-b	19-d	21-c
2-b	6-a	10-c	14-a	18-a	20-a	22-b
3-a	7-d	11-d	15-d			
4-d	8-b	12-b	16-c			

TEST 1

1-c	16-b	31-a	46-c	61-b	76-a	91-a
2-b	17-b	32-c	47-d	62-a	77-b	92-c
3-a	18-a	33-d	48-c	63-c	78-c	93-b
4-d	19-c	34-b	49-b	64-d	79-d	94-c
5-d	20-b	35-a	50-d	65-c	80-a	95-b
6-a	21-d	36-d	51-c	66-a	81-c	96-a
7-a	22-a	37-c	52-a	67-c	82-d	97-c
8-d	23-c	38-c	53-b	68-a	83-c	98-b
9-b	24-a	39-b	54-d	69-d	84-a	99-d
10-a	25-c	40-d	55-c	70-c	85-b	100-a
11-c	26-d	41-c	56-a	71-b	86-c	
12-b	27-c	42-a	57-b	72-a	87-d	
13-d	28-b	43-b	58-c	73-b	88-a	
14-a	29-c	44-c	59-a	74-c	89-c	
15-b	30-a	45-a	60-d	75-d	90-d	

TEST 2

1-b	16-d	31-b	46-c	61-a	76-d	91-d
2-c	17-b	32-a	47-d	62-d	77-a	92-a
3-d	18-a	33-d	48-b	63-b	78-c	93-b
4-b	19-b	34-b	49-c	65-c	79-a	94-a
5-b	20-c	35-c	50-a	65-a	80-c	95-c
6-c	21-d	36-a	51-b	66-d	81-b	96-d
7-a	22-b	37-b	52-d	67-a	82-a	97-b
8-c	23-a	38-d	53-c	68-c	83-c	98-a
9-b	24-c	39-c	54-a	69-b	84-a	99-c
10-d	25-d	40-a	55-c	70-c	85-d	100-a
11-c	26-c	41-b	56-b	71-a	86-c	
12-a	27-a	42-c	57-d	72-b	87-a	
13-b	28-b	43-d	58-a	73-a	88-b	
14-c	29-d	44-b	59-b	74-c	89-c	
15-b	30-c	45-a	60-c	75-b	90-b	

26. Circulation is increased by the use of:
    a) joint movement for toes
    b) effleurage
    c) joint movement for foot
    d) thumb compression   D

27. Thumb compression should be avoided in an area where a physician has removed a/an:
    a) plantar's wart
    b) ingrown toenail
    c) nail fungus
    d) mole   A

28. Flexibility is promoted by this technique:
    a) thumb compression
    b) effleurage
    c) metatarsal scissors
    d) fist twist   C

29. Fist twist compression is a friction movement which requires:
    a) great concentration
    b) deep rubbing
    c) gentleness
    d) many applications   B

30. The tapotement movements used to end a massage are commonly known as:
    a) final effleurage
    b) tapping touches
    c) tingle toes
    d) percussion movements   D

Chapter 12

NAIL TIPS

1. A nail tip is an artificial nail made of any of the following, EXCEPT:
   a) plastic
   b) rubber
   c) nylon
   d) acetate

   B

2. Tips are adhered to the natural nail to give the client's nails added:
   a) strength
   b) wells
   c) length
   d) buffers

   C

3. A tip worn with no overlay is very:
   a) beautiful
   b) weak
   c) strong
   d) long

   B

4. A tip with no overlay is considered a:
   a) temporary service
   b) finished nail
   c) unfinished nail
   d) natural look

   A

5. To smooth the natural nail and remove the shine, you should use an:
   a) adhesive
   b) antibacterial agent
   c) alcohol sanitizer
   d) abrasive

   D

6. The point of contact for the artificial nail tip and the natural nail plate is called the:
   a) extension
   b) glue
   c) well
   d) bed

   C

7. Tip wells are full or:
   a) quarter
   b) half
   c) three-quarters
   d) three-eighths

   B

8. The artificial nail tip should never cover more than this amount of the natural nail plate:
   a) $\frac{1}{2}$
   b) $\frac{1}{3}$
   c) $\frac{2}{3}$
   d) $\frac{3}{4}$

   B

9. Before receiving a nail tip application, the client should wash her hands with:
   a) alcohol
   b) antibacterial soap
   c) fungicide
   d) lanolin

   B

10. Buff the nail plate to remove:
    a) soap residue
    b) nail polish
    c) dust
    d) natural oil

    D

11. Properly sized tips will cover the nail plate from:
    a) lunula to free edge
    b) sidewall to sidewall
    c) lunula to mid-nail
    d) free edge out

    B

12. Nail tip procedures are worked starting with the:
    a) little finger, right hand
    b) thumb, left hand
    c) little finger, left hand
    d) thumb, right hand

    C

13. If you accidentally touch the client's nails after you apply antiseptic, you must prepare them again by:
    a) swabbing with alcohol
    b) reapplying antiseptic
    c) washing with formalin
    d) cleaning again, reapply antiseptic

    D

14. Adhesive is applied to the:
    a) nail plate
    b) lunula
    c) cuticle area
    d) free edge

    A

15. To help prevent trapped air bubbles in adhesive, the adhesive may be applied to the:
    a) free edge of tip
    b) sidewall
    c) well of tip
    d) spatula

    C

16. In sliding on tips, find stop against the free edge at:
    a) 33° angle
    b) 45° angle
    c) 50° angle
    c) 55° angle

    B

17. Hold the tip in place until dry for:
    a) 3 to 4 seconds
    b) 5 to 10 seconds
    c) 12 to 15 seconds
    d) 15 to 20 seconds

    B

18. A bead of adhesive is applied to the seam between the natural nail plate and the tip to:
    a) add beauty
    b) strengthen stress points
    c) add length
    d) smooth ridges

    B

19. Artificial nail tips should not be trimmed straight across, as this will cause the plastic to:
    a) weaken
    b) lift
    c) crack
    d) break

    A

20. To blend the artificial tip with the natural nail, you should:
    a) use extra adhesive
    b) use trimmers
    c) gently file and buff
    d) cover nail with tip

    C

21. A tip should blend with the natural nail so there is no:
    a) air bubble
    b) excess adhesive
    c) jagged edge
    d) visible line

    D

22. A nail tip should be covered with:
    a) wrap, acrylic or gel nail
    b) two base coats
    c) three polish coats
    d) nail strengthener base coat

    A

23. Clients who want temporary tips need a:
    a) quick manicure
    b) two-appointment service
    c) three-appointment service
    d) four-appointment service

    B

24. Clients wearing tips need to come back to the salon for service:
    a) weekly
    b) monthly
    c) biannually
    d) yearly

    A

25. During weekly maintenance, tips should be:
    a) clipped shorter
    b) removed and reapplied
    c) reglued at seam
    d) sanitized

    C

26. To remove polish on nail tips, use a/an:
    a) acetone remover
    b) buffer block
    c) cuticle remover
    d) non-acetone remover

    D

27. Never nip off artificial nail tips, as you might cause damage to the:
   a) natural free edge   c) nail bed
   b) nail root   d) cuticle   C

28. To remove artificial nail tips, use glue remover or:
   a) buffer block   c) emery board
   b) acetone   d) steel pusher   B

29. After soaking in remover, softened tips are carefully removed using a/an:
   a) steel pusher   c) nail clipper
   b) emery board   d) orangewood stick D

30. To remove glue residue from natural nail, use a/an:
   a) fine buffer block   c) orangewood stick
   b) cuticle oil   d) cuticle remover   A

NAIL WRAPS

Chapter 13

1. Nail wraps are sometimes called:
   - a) tips
   - b) overlays
   - c) gel nails
   - d) bonded nails

   B

2. Nail wraps are used on natural nails or artificial tips to:
   - a) provide base for polish
   - b) hide poor technical work
   - c) repair or strengthen
   - d) provide base for nail art

   C

3. Overlays are bonded to the front of the:
   - a) nail plate
   - b) free edge
   - c) lunula
   - d) skin under free edge

   A

4. When adhesive is applied to a silk wrap, the wrap becomes:
   - a) strong
   - b) smooth
   - c) wrinkled
   - d) transparent

   D

5. The linen wrap must be covered with colored polish because it is:
   - a) closely woven
   - b) opaque
   - c) heavy
   - d) transparent

   B

6. Polish remover causes paper wraps to:
   - a) rip
   - b) become brittle
   - c) dissolve
   - d) turn yellow

   C

7. The pointed applicator tip on nail adhesive is called a/an:
   - a) extender tip
   - b) bonding tip
   - c) spatula tip
   - d) cuticle tip

   A

8. Nail wrap procedures begin on the:
   - a) little finger, right hand
   - b) thumb, right hand
   - c) litter finger, left hand
   - d) thumb, left hand

   C

9. The adhesive is applied to all ten nails on the:
   - a) free edge
   - b) entire surface
   - c) lunula
   - d) sidewall

   B

10. Trimming fabric slightly smaller than nail plate prevents fabric from:
    - a) shrinking
    - b) stretching
    - c) raveling
    - d) lifting

    D

11. The final two adhesive applications in a fabric wrap are applied:
    - a) over fabric
    - b) under fabric
    - c) to cuticle
    - d) 10 minutes apart

    A

12. To clean adhesive extender tips, soak in acetone and then poke hole with a clean:
    - a) cotton swab
    - b) pipe cleaner
    - c) orangewood stick
    - d) toothpick

    D

13. To acquaint clients with the latest manicure looks, host:
    - a) manicure lessons
    - b) a cosmetics party
    - c) a nail fashion night
    - d) a fund-raiser event

    C

14. Offer clients a nailcare fashion kit with a gift certificate and:
    a) nail polish
    b) trial-sized products
    c) hand cream
    d) emery boards

    B

15. Fabric wraps are maintained after two weeks with a:
    a) glue fill
    b) polish change
    c) water manicure
    d) fabric fill

    A

16. In a glue fill, adhesive is applied first to the:
    a) free edge
    b) entire nail
    c) new nail growth
    d) edges of nail wrap

    C

17. A purpose of applying adhesive to the entire nail in a glue fill is to:
    a) smooth ridges
    b) reseal wrap
    c) apply new wrap
    d) form base for polish

    B

18. In a four week fabric wrap maintenance visit, the new nail growth is:
    a) covered with fabric
    b) polished
    c) ignored
    d) measured

    A

19. A strip of fabric cut to 1/8 inch is called a:
    a) repair patch
    b) fabric wrap
    c) center application
    d) stress strip

    D

20. A piece of fabric cut to completely cover a crack or break in the nail is called a:
    a) repair patch
    b) fabric wrap
    c) complete application
    d) stress strip

    A

21. The lightweight tissue paper used in wraps is called:
    a) wrapping paper
    b) mending tissue
    c) liquid paper
    d) onionskin

    B

22. The heavy adhesive used in paper wraps is called:
    a) paste
    b) glue
    c) liquid nails
    d) mending liquid

    D

23. Paper wraps are used to give a nail:
    a) length
    b) regrowth area
    c) strength
    d) base for nail art

    C

24. Paper wraps are not recommended for nails which are:
    a) short
    b) extra long
    c) pointed
    d) square

    B

25. When fitting the tissue, the edges should be:
    a) feathered
    b) straight
    c) curved
    d) past the sidewall

    A

26. In applying a paper wrap, the mending tissue should be tucked:
    a) around sidewall
    b) at nail plate center
    c) under free edge
    d) at lunula

    C

27. After smoothing applied tissue, the top and free edge of the nail should be covered with two or three coats of:
    a) mending liquid
    b) acrylic
    c) base coat
    d) top coat

    A

28. Before applying polish, the paper wrap's surface should be smoothed by applying:
   a) base coat
   b) ridge filler
   c) mending liquid
   d) buffing compound

   B

29. A polish made up of tiny fibers to strengthen and preserve the natural nail is:
   a) nail strengthener
   b) base coat
   c) liquid nail wrap
   d) top coat

   C

30. Liquid nail wrap is applied to the nail by:
   a) spray
   b) spatula
   c) soaking in it
   d) brush

   D

ACRYLIC NAILS

chapter 14

1. Acrylic nails are also known as:
   a) nail tips
   b) sculptured nails
   c) plastic nails
   d) hard nails

   B

2. Acrylic nails are made by combining two acrylic products, one liquid and one:
   a) powdered
   b) soft
   c) gel
   d) preformed

   A

3. Acrylic nails can be applied to all the following EXCEPT:
   a) natural nails
   b) nail tips
   c) paper wraps
   d) nail forms

   C

4. Something made up of many small molecules that are not attached to one another is called a:
   a) catalyst
   b) polymerization
   c) polymer
   d) monomer

   D

5. Molecules attached in long chains, usually forming something hard, are called:
   a) polymers
   b) monomers
   c) catalysts
   d) curers

   A

6. An ingredient which speeds up a process is called a:
   a) monomer
   b) polymer
   c) catalyst
   d) curing agent

   C

7. The one-color acrylic process produces a nail that is usually worn:
   a) by models
   b) with polish
   c) very long
   d) on special occasions

   B

8. The two-color acrylic nail method produces a nail that is usually worn:
   a) natural nail
   b) silk wrap
   c) French Manicure
   d) linen wrap

   C

9. Acrylic powder is available in all the following colors EXCEPT:
   a) clear
   b) pink
   c) white
   d) red

   D

10. The product applied to the natural nail so the acrylic product will adhere is the:
    a) primer
    b) acrylic liquid
    c) acrylic powder
    d) nail form

    A

11. The product which chemically dissolves nooks and crannies into the natural nail for better acrylic application is called:
    a) acrylic liquid
    b) non-etching primer
    c) etching primer
    d) abrasive

    C

12. Plastic gloves and safety glasses should always be worn when working with:
   a) primers
   b) abrasives
   c) acrylic powders
   d) acrylic liquids

   A

13. The soft balls of acrylic are applied to the nail with:
   a) tweezers
   b) an application tube
   c) a sable brush
   d) an orangewood stick

   C

14. The nail form should be positioned so that it fits snugly, and the natural nail free edge is:
   a) under the form
   b) butted to form edge
   c) $1/16$ inch away
   d) over the form

   D

15. Primer should dry on nail until the color is:
   a) yellow
   b) chalky white
   c) pink
   d) bright white

   B

16. To form an acrylic ball, the sable brush is dipped into:
   a) liquid, then powder
   b) powder, then liquid
   c) powder, liquid, powder
   d) liquid, powder, liquid

   A

17. Touching the primed area of the nail with a wet brush prior to acrylic application will cause the acrylic to:
   a) be contaminated
   b) harden rapidly
   c) separate
   d) lift

   D

18. In acrylic application, the first acrylic ball is used to form the:
   a) nail plate
   b) free edge
   c) entire nail
   d) sidewalls

   B

19. Acrylic should be applied by using this brush technique:
   a) dab and press
   b) paint stroke
   c) "x"-pattern'
   d) dot, then paint

   A

20. For a natural-looking nail, acrylic application near cuticle, sidewall and free edge should be:
   a) $1/16$ inch away
   b) moderately thick
   c) extremely thin
   d) white powder

   C

21. Acrylic nails are dry when gentle tapping with brush handle produces a:
   a) chip
   b) hollow ring
   c) scratch
   d) clicking sound

   D

22. To look their best, one-step acrylic nails should have a weekly:
   a) fill
   b) water manicure
   c) buffing
   d) removal

   B

23. All acrylic nails need maintenance every:
   a) day
   b) week
   c) two to three weeks
   d) two months

   C

24. To smooth out imperfections when applying the final acrylic beads, the brush should:
   a) glide
   b) be wet
   c) be dry
   d) be new

   A

25. When applying acrylic nail over bitten natural nail, before applying form you must create:
    a) long free edge
    b) new color powder
    c) bite preventative
    d) part of nail plate

    D

26. The addition of acrylic to the new growth area of the nails is called:
    a) crack repair
    b) rebalancing
    c) lift
    d) polishing

    B

27. Without new growth rebalancing acrylic maintenance, the area near the cuticle, in comparison to the rest of the nail, will be:
    a) lower
    b) whiter
    c) pinker
    d) higher

    A

28. The addition of acrylic to reinforce the nail and fill a crack is called:
    a) fill-in
    b) strengthening
    c) crack repair
    d) buffing

    C

29. Attempting acrylic removal with nippers can seriously damage natural nail:
    a) free edge
    b) plate
    c) cuticle
    d) root

    B

30. Acrylic products which do not smell as strongly as traditional acrylic products are called:
    a) old
    b) contaminated
    c) polymers
    d) odorless

    D

31. When odorless nails are dry, the surface will feel:
    a) tacky
    b) smooth
    c) rough
    d) oil

    A

32. For the holidays, create packages with different product combinations and sizes priced from:
    a) $3 to $5
    b) $5 to $15
    c) $15 to $20
    d) $20 to $25

    B

GELS

1. Strong, durable artificial nails which are brushed on the nail plate like polish are called:
   - a) sculptured nails
   - b) gel nails
   - c) nail strengtheners
   - d) primer

   B

2. An ultraviolet light or a halogen light is required to harden:
   - a) light-cured gels
   - b) nail strengthener
   - c) acrylic nails
   - d) base coat

   A

3. No-light gels harden when a gel activator is applied, or when nails are soaked in:
   - a) fungicide
   - b) acetone
   - c) alcohol
   - d) water

   D

4. Colored gels make a good base for:
   - a) nail tips
   - b) acrylic nails
   - c) nail art
   - d) top coat

   C

5. Gel is applied by brushing on to:
   - a) free edge
   - b) entire nail
   - c) lunula
   - d) cuticle

   B

6. To prevent hardening of gel during procedure, keep brush and gel away from:
   - a) curing light
   - b) acetone
   - c) alcohol
   - d) cold air

   A

7. A properly applied second coat of gel has the appearance of a/an:
   - a) acrylic nail
   - b) cuticle oil
   - c) nail tip
   - d) glossy top coat

   D

8. Gel nail residue should be removed with:
   - a) water
   - b) acetone
   - c) alcohol
   - d) hand lotion

   C

9. Inadequately shielded ultraviolet lamps can damage:
   - a) eyes
   - b) gel
   - c) cuticle
   - d) acrylic

   A

10. Gel nails over forms are the best choice for clients who want length without:
    - a) strength
    - b) color
    - c) weight
    - d) shape

    C

11. To create gel nails over forms, gel must be applied several times, usually:
    - a) three
    - b) four
    - c) five
    - d) six

    B

12. No-light gel activator is also called a/an:
    - a) adhesive dryer
    - b) heat activator
    - c) nail antiseptic
    - d) water cure

    A

13. With no-light gels, a second application of gel is often:
    - a) time-consuming
    - b) dangerous
    - c) messy
    - d) unnecessary

    D

14. Gel nails should be maintained every:
    a) week
    b) two to three weeks
    c) two to three months
    d) month

B

15. Gel nails are removed by soaking nails in gel remover or:
    a) hydrogen peroxide
    b) alcohol
    c) acetone
    d) water

C

THE CREATIVE TOUCH

chapter 16

1. To promote nail art to your clients, you should:
   a) wear it yourself
   b) practice
   c) take classes
   d) buy an airbrush ____

2. To give sparkle to a nail art design, use:
   a) glitter
   b) gems
   c) sequins
   d) metallic polish ____

3. To adhere gems to nail, put on:
   a) natural nail
   b) with glue
   c) while top coat's tacky
   d) with acrylic ____

4. To seal gem to nail, cover entire nail, including gems, with:
   a) acrylic liquid
   b) top coat
   c) gel nail
   d) spray adhesive ____

5. If the silver backing comes off a gem, it cannot be reused due to its inability to:
   a) resist germs
   b) add texture
   c) stick
   d) reflect color ____

6. Lines in nail art are easy to create using:
   a) striping tape
   b) forms
   c) narrow brushes
   d) black polish ____

7. Striping tape is applied to a nail which is:
   a) sculptured
   b) polished and wet
   c) polished and dry
   d) natural and buffed ____

8. Fragile leafing available in gold, silver, and copper is called:
   a) leaf
   b) foil
   c) leading
   d) nail strengthener ____

9. Both striping tape an foil are sealed to the nail by being covered with:
   a) liquid gel nail
   b) acrylic liquid
   c) glue
   d) top coat ____

10. When applying clear polish over a nail painting, be sure the brush is wet enough in order to avoid:
    a) smearing the painting
    b) losing brush hairs
    c) a smudged top coat
    d) air bubbles ____

11. The most popular technique used in airbrushing is:
    a) the sweep
    b) marbling
    c) the French Manicure
    d) striping ____

12. In order to draw with an airbrush you must use:
    a) extra paint
    b) a design tool
    c) an adhesive
    d) sponges ____

13. Begin practicing use of an airbrush on:
    a) absorbent paper
    b) your own nails
    c) styrofoam
    d) tissues ____

14. Most people use an airbrush at what distance from the nail surface?
    a) one to two inches c) three to four inches
    b) two to three inches d) four to five inches ____

15. After applying one to two coats of protective airbrush nail glaze, all nails need to dry for:
    a) 3 minutes c) 10 minutes
    b) 7 minutes d) 12 minutes ____

16. The color fade can only be accomplished with an airbrush because the color changes with no:
    a) bump or line c) smudges
    b) air bubbles d) lengthy delays ____

17. To add shimmer to a French beige manicure paint, mist over it with:
    a) gold highlight c) silver highlight
    b) water d) sparkles ____

SALON BUSINESS

Chapter 17

1. The nail care industry annually does business of:
   a) $1 million   c) $2 billion
   b) $5 million   d) $6 billion   _C_

2. The average full-service salon employs this many nail technicians:
   a) one   c) five
   b) three   d) seven   _A_

3. A disadvantage of full-service salons for the nail technician is:
   a) hair care   c) not enough clients
   b) skin care   d) no backup when gone _D_

4. In a nails-only salon, you have the opportunity to interact with other technicians as well as the potential to:
   a) increase your business   c) breathe toxic fumes   _A_
   b) be exposed to germs   d) have competition

5. To develop experience in creative artificial nail services, a technician should consider:
   a) entering contests   c) working in full-
                                  service salon   _B_
   b) working in nails-only salon d) art classes

6. To evaluate if a salon's working environment is right for you, you should consider all the following EXCEPT:
   a) continuing education   c) owner's hairstyle
      opportunities
   b) salon's reputation   d) how you will be paid _C_

7. Medical, life and liability insurances are examples of employee:
   a) risk   c) expenses
   b) benefits   d) rights   _B_

8. The money you make is called:
   a) income   c) taxes
   b) expenses   d) tips   _A_

9. The money you spend is called:
   a) allowance   c) withholding
   b) outcome   d) expenses   _D_

10. Income includes all the following EXCEPT:
    a) salary   c) withholding
    b) commissions   d) tips   _C_

11. Your expenses working in a salon could include all the following EXCEPT:
    a) car repair   c) supplies
    b) equipment   d) professional books/
                          magazines   _A_

12. In order to be more efficient, you should record each day's schedule in a:
    a) master salon appointment book
    b) tax record book
    c) computer
    d) personal appointment calendar   *D*

13. To help keep accurate financial records, most salons use a/an:
    a) erasable ink pen
    b) accounting service
    c) honor system
    d) duplicate receipt book   *B*

14. Daily sales slips, appointment books and petty cash records are usually kept on file for:
    a) one year
    b) five years
    c) ten years
    d) twenty years   *A*

15. The payroll book, cancelled checks, monthly and yearly records and service and inventory records are used in filing tax returns, and are normally kept for at least:
    a) two years
    b) five years
    c) seven years
    d) ten years   *C*

16. Monthly and yearly records can be a valuable resource for:
    a) sheltering income
    b) determining peak and slow months
    c) buying supplies
    d) raising prices   *B*

17. Daily inventory records help to quickly detect loss of supplies and retail product due to:
    a) theft
    b) heat
    c) cold
    d) expiration dates   *A*

18. The income you make minus all your expenses is called:
    a) gross pay
    b) withholding
    c) tax deferred
    d) net income   *D*

19. Records to help compare use of supplies with services are called:
    a) inventory
    b) material and supply levels
    c) client service records
    d) retail receipts   *B*

20. The listing of services rendered and products sold to each client is called the:
    a) material level
    b) inventory record
    c) client service record
    d) gross income   *C*

21. Supplies used in providing services are:
    a) consumption supplies
    b) retail supplies
    c) business losses
    d) ordered daily   *A*

22. Keeping an accurate record of appointments reduces:
    a) supply waste
    b) paperwork
    c) retail theft
    d) overbooking appointments   *D*

23. Proper phone etiquette includes:
    a) answering promptly
    b) making clients hold
    c) answering only after six rings
    d) talking in slang   *A*

24. When scheduling an appointment, be sure to get the client's:
    a) polish preference
    b) credit card number
    c) name and phone number
    d) driver's license number   *C*

25. To avoid a scheduling error, when taking telephone appointments you should:
   a) never take phone calls
   b) repeat information to client
   c) allow time between appointments
   d) call client back

   B

26. To reduce the number of no-shows, it is a good idea to:
   a) call clients to confirm
   b) overbook
   c) charge for missed appointments
   d) cancel if client is late

   A

27. To conclude your service, always ask clients if they:
   a) will pay cash
   b) wear rubber gloves
   c) bite their nails
   d) would like another appointment

   D

28. Call your clients to alert them if you are running late by more than:
   a) 10 minutes
   b) 15 minutes
   c) 20 minutes
   d) 30 minutes

   B

29. A written description of services and prices is called the:
   a) service contract
   b) service list
   c) referral brochure
   d) job description

   B

30. A pricing practice to be avoided is the offering of reduced prices:
   a) to attract clientele
   b) to promote a service
   c) to only selected clients
   d) in a package deal

   C

SELLING NAIL PRODUCTS AND SERVICES

Chapter 18

1. Successful nail technicians are skilled professionals and:
   a) very artistic
   b) good at bookkeeping
   c) good salespeople
   d) salon managers

   _C_

2. One of the basic steps in selling is to:
   a) talk fast
   b) know the product
   c) wave hands around
   d) offer smallest size

   _B_

3. A specific fact about a product or service is called a:
   a) feature
   b) cost base
   c) service point
   d) profit center

   _A_

4. How a product will fulfill your client's needs is called a:
   a) service point
   b) feature
   c) personal chemistry
   d) benefit

   _D_

5. The best nail choice for a cosmetics salesperson may be:
   a) short and polished
   b) medium and buffed
   c) long acrylic
   d) short gel

   _C_

6. The best nail choice for a pianist may be:
   a) short and natural-looking
   b) medium and polished
   c) long acrylic
   d) medium gel with artwork

   _A_

7. A client whose hands are frequently in water should not have:
   a) bright polish
   b) long tips
   c) top coat
   d) fabric wraps

   _D_

8. For special occasions, a client may want to match nails with:
   a) hairstyle
   b) clothing
   c) makeup
   d) pedicure

   _B_

9. One way to sell products is to tell clients about them:
   a) while you work
   b) after they've paid
   c) when scheduling appointment
   d) when they ask

   _A_

10. To generate interest in your services, prominently display your:
    a) resume
    b) pedicure foot baths
    c) service list
    d) beauty school diploma

    _C_

11. To encourage retail sales, offer your clients all the following EXCEPT:
    a) product brochures
    b) product attractively displayed
    c) free samples
    d) coffee and cookies

    _D_

12. You should sell your clients the products they need for:
    a) home acrylic application
    b) home nail maintenance
    c) home gel application
    d) home fabric wrap application

    B

13. A great way to sell retail products is to group those products in:
    a) pre-made packages
    b) several price ranges
    c) the top shelf of your area
    d) a, b & c

    A

14. A package could contain products needed to:
    a) maintain a French Manicure
    b) airbrush at home
    c) apply linen wraps
    d) apply nail tape

    A

15. If you don't know the answer to a client's question:
    a) pretend that you do
    b) change the subject
    c) refer them to another technician
    d) volunteer to find out

    D

16. A client's objection should be answered:
    a) by talking rapidly
    b) rudely
    c) honestly and pleasantly
    d) with sarcasm

    c

17. When a client has valid objections to a product or service, you should:
    a) walk away
    b) suggest another option
    c) get angry
    d) refuse them service

    B

18. When a client decides to buy a product or service, you have:
    a) closed the sale
    b) out-smarted them
    c) pleased the boss
    d) successfully maneuvered them

    A

19. Suggesting products or services for clients to buy is called:
    a) being pushy
    b) retailing
    c) final service
    d) suggestion selling

    D

20. You will be successful at suggestion selling when you can match products and services with your client's:
    a) needs and wants
    b) budget
    c) clothing
    d) hairstyle

    A

21. When a client makes another appointment, give them a "reminder card" by writing the date and time on your:
    a) scratch pad
    b) 3" x 5" card
    c) business card
    d) pink reminder papers

    C

22. Advance scheduling is a good way to:
    a) plan days off
    b) build steady clientele
    c) plan budgets
    d) order supplies

    B

TYPICAL STATE EXAMINATIONS

100 MULTIPLE CHOICE QUESTIONS

Directions: Carefully read each statement. Insert on the blank line after each statement the letter representing the word or phrase that correctly completes the statement.

1. Ultraviolet radiation is harmful to:
   a) bones
   b) nail polish
   c) eyes
   d) acrylic tips   _C_

2. Liquid acrylic is a type of:
   a) polymer
   b) monomer
   c) catalyst
   d) curing   _B_

3. A condition in which white spots appear on the nails is called:
   a) leukonychia
   b) atrophy
   c) nevus
   d) super atrophy   _A_

4. State regulators expect a salon environment to be:
   a) sterile
   b) infectious
   c) decorative
   d) sanitary   _D_

5. By understanding body structure, you will be more proficient when doing:
   a) fiber wraps
   b) basic manicures
   c) pedicures
   d) hand & arm massage   _D_

6. All living things are made up of this basic unit, called the:
   a) cell
   b) protein
   c) nucleus
   d) beta blocker   _A_

7. Bacteria can be found nearly everywhere; there are this many known types:
   a) 15,000
   b) 5,000
   c) 10,000
   d) 1,500   _A_

8. This activity is dangerous around nail chemicals:
   a) gossiping
   b) chewing gum
   c) talking loudly
   d) smoking   _D_

9. This medical specialty focuses on skin problems:
   a) cardiology
   b) dermatology
   c) esthetics
   d) podiatry   _B_

10. A client consultation is the conversation you have with the client before:
    a) starting the service
    b) they make appointment
    c) they pay
    d) they buy retail products   _A_

11. The manicure table should have a bulb of this wattage in the lamp:
    a) 60
    c) 40
    b) 100
    d) 150

    _a_

12. Natural immunity is obtained by keeping the body:
    a) warm
    c) underweight
    b) healthy
    d) overweight

    _B_

13. The condition in which the nail loosens from the nail bed is:
    a) paronychia
    c) onychia
    b) oncophagy
    d) onycholysis

    _D_

14. Sculptured nails are also known as:
    a) acrylic nails
    c) nail wraps
    b) manicured nails
    d) extra long nails

    _A_

15. The recommended maintenance schedule for all acrylic nails is every:
    a) month
    c) day
    b) two to three weeks
    d) six months

    _B_

16. Your sense of right and wrong when you interact with clients, employer and coworkers is called:
    a) honesty
    c) moral values
    b) professional ethics
    d) moodiness

    _B_

17. Massage, nerve impulses and light rays are some of the ways to stimulate:
    a) phalanges
    c) sanitation
    b) muscles
    d) eyes

    _B_

18. The muscles which can cause goose bumps are called the:
    a) arrector pili
    c) goosli muscles
    b) papillae
    d) lesion

    _A_

19. An emery board is an example of an item that is:
    a) wet sanitized
    c) disposable
    b) heat sanitized
    d) purchased individually

    _C_

20. If the nail tip covers the nail plate from sidewall to sidewall, it is:
    a) too wide
    c) too long
    b) properly sized
    d) too narrow

    _B_

21. The French Manicure look can be created through the:
    a) one-color acrylic method
    c) proper buffing techniques
    b) proper diet
    d) two-color acrylic method

    _D_

22. In acrylic applications, the free edge is formed with the:
    a) first acrylic ball
    c) nail file
    b) third acrylic ball
    d) second acrylic ball

    _A_

23. Soaking in water hardens:
    a) acrylic balls
    c) no-light gels
    b) rhinestone applications
    d) acrylic residue

    _C_

24. Soft or fragile nails should be filed using a/an:
    a) emery board
    c) chamois buffer
    b) metal nail file
    d) nail brush

    _A_

25. Hypoallergenic products are used for the client's:
    a) pharmacist
    b) skin cancer
    c) safety
    d) acne

    C

26. The movements of the body are controlled by the:
    a) efferent nerves
    b) peripheral system
    c) blood
    d) central nervous system

    D

27. When conditions are unfavorable for reproduction, bacteria will go dormant after forming a tough covering called a:
    a) shell
    b) mitosis
    c) spore
    d) flagella

    C

28. Non-acetone remover is used to remove polish from:
    a) hangnails
    b) artificial tips
    c) toenails
    d) accidental spills on clothing

    B

29. A repair patch is a piece of fabric cut to:
    a) nail's shape
    b) look like a daisy
    c) completely cover crack or break
    d) 1/2 inch by 1/2 inch

    C

30. Insomnia, watery eyes and sluggishness are symptoms of chemical:
    a) overexposure
    b) inhalation
    c) burn
    d) poisoning

    A

31. In order to have a good working relationship with coworkers, you should:
    a) respect their opinions
    b) use deodorant
    c) buy their lunch
    d) point out mistakes

    A

32. Liquid nail wrap is used to:
    a) speed silk wrap procedure
    b) preserve nail art
    c) strengthen natural nail
    d) cover fungi

    C

33. The opaqueness of linen wraps requires that they be covered with:
    a) glitter
    b) mending tissue
    c) clear polish
    d) colored polish

    D

34. Always refuse service and refer a client to a physician if they have a skin or nail:
    a) hangnail
    b) inflammation
    c) bruise
    d) callus

    B

35. Tanning is caused by exposing skin to the sun's:
    a) ultraviolet rays
    b) keratoma
    c) vitamin D
    d) carotene

    A

36. Learning about other services offered at the salon, such as hair and skin care, and then telling your clients about them, is called salon:
    a) performance
    b) showoff
    c) networking
    d) promotion

    D

37. The hardening process in acrylic nails is known as:
    a) catalyst
    b) polymerization
    c) curing
    d) monomer

    C

38. The best way to protect yourself and your clients against infection is to always:
   a) ask if they have an infection
   b) wear masks
   c) sanitize implements properly
   d) sit at arm's length   *C*

39. Mending liquid is a heavy adhesive used to apply:
   a) silk wraps
   b) paper wraps
   c) linen wraps
   d) nail gems   *B*

40. After removing an artificial nail, any remaining glue residue is removed by using a/an:
   a) emery board
   b) oily remover
   c) steel pusher
   d) fine buffer block   *D*

41. The technical name for callus is:
   a) freckle
   b) stratum lucidum
   c) keratoma
   d) mole   *C*

42. Bacilli and spirilla propel themselves with hairlike projections known as:
   a) flagella
   b) propellants
   c) mitosis
   d) cocci   *A*

43. To protect hands and nails when doing housework, clients should wear:
   a) silicone lotion
   b) rubber gloves
   c) clear polish
   d) dust mask   *B*

44. Linen wraps are the:
   a) hardest to do
   b) easiest to rip or tear
   c) most popular wrap
   d) hardest to maintain   *C*

45. The nerve which supplies impulses to the top of the foot is the:
   a) dorsal
   b) digital
   c) saphenous
   d) ulnar   *A*

46. Unsanitary implements can cause these nail disorders:
   a) onychomycosis
   b) mold
   c) onychia and paronychia
   d) nevus   *C*

47. Cuticle pushers are also known as:
   a) nippers
   b) oils
   c) emery boards
   d) steel pushers   *D*

48. The most common nail shape for male clients is:
   a) square
   b) oval
   c) round
   d) pointed   *C*

49. To prevent contamination of the disinfectant, disinfection containers should be kept:
   a) warm
   b) covered
   c) cold
   d) in cupboards   *B*

50. Client service records are usually kept on:
   a) pink paper
   b) blue paper
   c) triplicate forms
   d) index cards   *D*

51. Foot files are used to remove:
   a) warts
   b) hangnails
   c) callus growths
   d) fungus   *C*

52. Eyes can be damaged by improperly shielded:
    a) ultraviolet lamps
    b) fingerbowls
    c) polish
    d) autoclaves

    A

53. The number of known elements is:
    a) 96
    b) 106
    c) 101
    d) 108

    B

54. An example of an employee benefit would be any of the following EXCEPT:
    a) medical insurance
    b) life insurance
    c) paid parking space
    d) earn minimum wage

    D

55. Your personal problems should always be:
    a) shared with coworkers
    b) shared with clients
    c) left at home
    d) told to the boss

    C

56. A client with athlete's foot may not receive:
    a) a pedicure
    b) foot massage
    c) colored polish
    d) pedicure slippers

    A

57. To draw with an airbrush, you need to use a/an:
    a) orangewood stick
    b) design tool
    c) sponge
    d) nail pen

    B

58. On an annual basis, the nail care industry annually does this much business:
    a) $3 billion
    b) $5 million
    c) $2 billion
    d) $10 million

    C

59. A common condition in which the cuticle around the nail splits is known as:
    a) hangnails
    b) skin overgrowth
    c) nail crack
    d) callus

    A

60. Prevent chemical accidents by never using a product if the container is not:
    a) sealed
    b) sanitized
    c) full
    d) labeled

    D

61. It is dangerous to judge if a chemical is safe by its:
    a) label
    b) odor
    c) ingredients
    d) MSDS

    B

62. Clear, white and pink are colors of:
    a) acrylic powder
    b) sable brushes
    c) toe separators
    d) paper towels

    A

63. The tacky feel of the surface of odorless acrylic nails indicates the nails are:
    a) old
    b) separating from nail plate
    c) dry
    d) needing a fill

    C

64. This layer of epidermis has cells that look like granules:
    a) stratum corneum
    b) stratum mucosum
    c) stratum lucidum
    d) stratum granulosum

    D

65. Nails which are thin, white and curved over the free edge are called:
    a) furrowed
    b) normal
    c) eggshell
    d) dry

    C

66. Color and gloss is added to the nail through the application of:
    a) colored polish
    b) silk wrap
    c) buffing compound
    d) mending liquid

    A

67. The appearance of a properly applied second coat of gel looks like:
    a) gelatin
    b) primer
    c) glossy top coat
    d) cuticle oil

    C

68. Formalin contains formaldehyde which causes the following EXCEPT:
    a) muscle pain
    b) lung irritation
    c) rash
    d) skin irritation

    A

69. To make them feel welcome, new clients should be:
    a) greeted by name
    b) given salon tour
    c) escorted to station
    d) all the above

    D

70. Most pedicure services are performed by starting with:
    a) right foot, little toe
    b) right foot, middle toe
    c) left foot, little toe
    d) left foot, big toe

    C

71. The client who wants length without weight should receive:
    a) paper wraps
    b) gel nails
    c) linen wraps
    d) silk wraps

    B

72. To give sparkle to a nail art design, use:
    a) gems
    b) metallic polish
    c) sequins
    d) fine buffer block

    A

73. If the nail or skin to be worked on is inflamed, broken, swollen or infected, the client must:
    a) be sanitized with alcohol
    b) be referred to a physician
    c) need a manicure
    d) scrub with soap

    B

74. Expenses are defined as the money you:
    a) earn
    b) save
    c) spend
    d) donate

    C

75. A technician who is a good salesperson and a skilled professional will also be:
    a) artistic
    b) good receptionist
    c) good manager
    d) very successful

    D

76. A client may want to match nails with clothing for a/an:
    a) special occasion
    b) few days
    c) few weeks
    d) entire year

    A

77. The "true skin" is the deep layer of skin which is called:
    a) cuticle
    b) cutis
    c) epidermis
    d) clavicle

    B

78. To remove gel nails, soak in acetone or:
    a) alcohol
    b) dishwashing liquid
    c) gel remover
    d) warm water

    C

79. If a chemical agent gets on your clothing, immediately:
    a) dab with water
    b) blot with towel
    c) use spot remover
    d) remove garment

    D

80. Natural nails can be lengthened by adding:
    a) artificial tips
    b) silk wraps
    c) paper wraps
    d) nail art

    A

81. A primer is applied to the natural nail in order for the acrylic product to:
a) dry properly   c) adhere
b) polish easily   d) prevent fungus _C_

82. A long acrylic nail may be the best choice for a woman who is a:
a) guitar player   c) gardener
b) pianist   d) cosmetic salesperson _D_

83. Dry cuticles can cause:
a) nail biting   c) hangnails
b) buffing problems   d) wraps to lift _C_

84. Most clients are relaxed by:
a) effleurage   c) thumb compression
b) clear polish applications d) metatarsal scissors _A_

85. Seven years is the amount of time you should keep business records which were used to:
a) pay off loans   c) pay employees
b) complete tax returns d) order supplies _B_

86. An acquired superficial, round and thickened patch of epidermis due to pressure or friction on the hands or feet is called:
a) cocci   c) keratoma
b) eczema   d) flagella _C_

87. Fabric wraps are not a good service choice for a client whose hands are frequently:
a) in gloves   c) photographed
b) held   d) in water _D_

88. Peak and slow months can be determined by reviewing your:
a) monthly records   c) customer list
b) tax withholding   d) supply inventory _A_

89. A liquid that kills or retards bacterial growth is a/an:
a) soap   c) antiseptic
b) solution   d) agent _C_

90. When applying acrylic over nail tips, you do not need to use a/an:
a) acrylic powder   c) acrylic liquid
b) sable brush   d) nail form _D_

91. Chemical storage should be in cool areas and away from:
a) appliance/furnace with pilot light c) perm solutions
b) hair colors   d) garbage cans _A_

92. To add shine to the nail, use a chamois buffer with pumice powder or:
a) water   c) dry polish
b) cuticle oil   d) cuticle remover _C_

93. An accounting service is often used to help salons keep:
a) making a profit   c) making loan payments
b) accurate financial records d) tax losses large _B_

94. A catalyst is an ingredient which causes a process to:
a) explode   c) speed up
b) slow down   d) remain static _C_

95. Sebum is secreted by:

a) seals   c) arteries

b) oil glands   d) infected skin   *B*

96. Plastic gloves and safety glasses should always be worn when working with:

a) primers   c) air brushes

b) gel nails   d) acrylic powders   *A*

97. The main part of the nail that is attached to the skin at the tip of the finger is the:

a) nail root   c) nail body

b) nail bed   d) nail fold   *C*

98. Skin's outer layer is called the:

a) dermis   c) subcutaneous tissue

b) epidermis   d) stratum corneum   *B*

99. The proper way to mix polish is to:

a) mix with top coat   c) tap bottle on table

b) shake vigorously   d) roll bottle between palms *D*

100. A weekly reconditioning hot oil manicure will benefit clients with:

a) dry cuticles   c) paper wraps

b) gel nails   d) arthritis   *A*

100 MULTIPLE CHOICE QUESTIONS

Directions: Carefully read each statement. Insert on the blank line after each statement the letter representing the word or phrase that correctly completes the statement.

1. Two-color acrylic application requires use of all the following EXCEPT:
a) white tip powder
c) pink powder
b) yellow powder
d) acrylic liquid   *B*

2. The common name for onychocryptosis is:
a) hangnail
c) ingrown nail
b) nail biting
d) bruise   *C*

3. Spraying nail antiseptic on nails removes:
a) cotton bits
c) nail filings
b) polish
d) natural oil   *D*

4. The HIV virus, which causes AIDS, may lay dormant in an infected person's system for up to:
a) 20 years
c) 50 years
b) 15 years
d) 3 years   *B*

5. The man's manicure procedure is always begun by working on the:
a) right hand
c) favored hand
b) left hand
d) nail filing   *B*

6. The chemicals from nail products enter your body in all these ways EXCEPT:
a) inhalation
c) injection
b) ingestion
d) skin contact   *C*

7. If pus is present, the skin or nail is:
a) infected
c) bruised
b) to be soaked in alcohol
d) inflamed   *A*

8. The technical name for athlete's foot is:
a) vitiligo
c) tinea pedis
b) chloasma
d) sarcoma   *C*

9. An important part of the consultation is to determine whether or not the home maintenance for a service fits the client's:
a) looks
c) budget
b) lifestyle
d) ability   *B*

10. Equipment is the term for items used in nail technology that are:
a) expensive
c) disposable
b) made of plastic
d) permanent   *D*

11. When pedicuring, the proper time to insert toe separators is before:
a) clipping nails
c) filing nails
b) polishing nails
d) soaking feet   *C*

12. The foot massage begins with:
    a) joint relaxer movements   c) metatarsal scissors
    b) thumb compression   d) brisk rubbing   *A*

13. Bacteria multiply at amazing speeds—in only half a day, a single bacteria cell can produce this many more:
    a) 6,000   c) 100,000
    b) 16 million   d) 25, 000   *B*

14. Albinism is the congenital absence of this substance from the body:
    a) albumin   c) melanin
    b) fungus   d) Vitamin C   *C*

15. Performing a service on an infected nail could cause your client a great deal of:
    a) healing   c) regrowth
    b) pain   d) filing   *B*

16. Phenolics are good for implement disinfection but are:
    a) difficult to work with   c) hard to find
    b) unbalanced   d) costly   *D*

17. Your best source of advertising to attract new clients is:
    a) radio   c) newspapers
    b) current satisfied clients   d) coupon mailers   *B*

18. A lamp bulb with high wattage will affect product performance when giving this service:
    a) sculptured nails   c) polish change
    b) gel nails   d) fiber wrap   *A*

19. The body is protected from harmful infection and bacteria through the white cells found in:
    a) urine   c) stress
    b) blood   d) white bread   *B*

20. A properly ventilated salon is one that vents fumes and vapors to the:
    a) reception area   c) outside
    b) bathroom   d) haircolor area   *C*

21. The difference between being a professional nail technician and "doing nails" is a good client:
    a) tip   c) location
    b) referral network   d) consultation   *D*

22. To avoid ingrown toenails, file the nails straight across with:
    a) steel implements   c) metal files
    b) slightly rounded corners   d) chamois buffers   *B*

23. Healthy nails result from:
    a) a general state of health   c) eating bananas
    b) regular trimming   d) drinking carrot juice   *A*

24. Fingernails grow faster than:
    a) hair   c) toenails
    b) bones   d) muscles   *C*

25. Paper wraps will dissolve in:
    a) water   c) polish applications
    b) dishwashing liquid   d) polish remover   *D*

26. To reseal wrap during a glue fill, apply adhesive to:
    a) any broken edges
    b) polish brush before application
    c) entire nail
    d) only thumb nails   *C*

27. Finished acrylic nails are:
    a) polymers
    b) monomers
    c) polymerizations
    d) catalysts   *A*

28. Foil leaf is available in gold, silver and:
    a) bronze
    b) copper
    c) turquoise
    d) onyx   *B*

29. Nonpathogenic bacteria belong to the group of bacteria known as:
    a) spirilla
    b) viruses
    c) cocci
    d) saprophytes   *D*

30. Problems or questions about your job should be discussed with:
    a) your butcher
    b) best friend
    c) your employer
    d) your mother   *C*

31. To ensure full potency, chemical agents for sanitation should be
    purchased:
    a) in bulk
    b) in small quantities
    c) by mail
    d) on sunny days   *B*

32. If no overlay is applied, an artificial tip is very:
    a) weak
    b) colorful
    c) ugly
    d) natural-looking   *A*

33. Light-cured gel nails are hardened using an ultraviolet light
    or a/an:
    a) non-acetone remover
    b) oily polish remover
    c) fungicide
    d) halogen light   *D*

34. Overlay is another name for:
    a) stencils
    b) nail wraps
    c) gem applications
    d) gel applications   *B*

35. The joints in the ankle and wrist are known as:
    a) ball joints
    b) cartilage
    c) gliding joints
    d) carpus   *C*

36. Extra long natural nails are not suited for this service:
    a) paper wraps
    b) reconditioning hot oil manicure
    c) French Manicure
    d) nail art   *A*

37. Percussion movements are also called:
    a) drum symphonies
    b) tapotement movements
    c) tingle toes
    d) tapping touches   *B*

38. In acrylic technique, when the sable brush is dipped into liquid,
    them powder, this forms:
    a) glue
    b) chalky white color
    c) baking soda
    d) an acrylic ball   *D*

39. Store acrylic products:
    a) on well-lit shelves
    b) near the manicure lamp
    c) in covered containers
    d) near a heating unit   *C*

40. An MSDS can be obtained from your salon's:
    a) distributor
    b) main office
    c) cleaning person
    d) fire department   *A*

41. The deep layer of skin is called the:
    a) epidermis
    b) dermis
    c) subcutaneous tissue
    d) nutrient level

    B

42. An orangewood stick is classified as a/an:
    a) nail file
    b) equipment
    c) implement
    d) reusable item

    C

43. The free edge of sculptured nails should be shaped with a/an:
    a) tweezer
    b) cuticle nipper
    c) chamois buffer
    d) metal nail file

    D

44. Striping tape is used to create lines when doing:
    a) football field markings
    b) nail art
    c) toenail clipping
    d) French Manicure

    B

45. Onychauxis is the technical term for a nail's:
    a) overgrowth
    b) infection
    c) bruise
    d) removal

    A

46. Chloasma is commonly known as:
    a) freckles
    b) birthmark
    c) liver spots
    d) tanning

    C

47. An accidental splash of solvent or primer can seriously injure the:
    a) nail
    b) polish
    c) implements
    d) eyes

    D

48. Manicure friction massage involves a wringing movement on the:
    a) toe
    b) arm
    c) fingers
    d) wrist

    B

49. When removing artificial tips, first soak them in remover to:
    a) dissolve free edge
    b) remove polish
    c) soften them
    d) dissolve sidewalls

    C

50. The chalky white color of primer during acrylic application indicates the primer is:
    a) dry
    b) odorless
    c) old
    d) not properly mixed

    A

51. A second coat of product is often unnecessary when applying:
    a) colored lacquer
    b) no-light gels
    c) light-cured gels
    d) acrylic nails

    B

52. The polish top coat should be tacky when these are applied:
    a) tips
    b) paper wraps
    c) gel nails
    d) gems

    D

53. Odorless acrylics are self-leveling, which means they require less:
    a) product
    b) brushing
    c) shaping
    d) buffing

    C

54. Consumable supplies are the supplies used to:
    a) provide services
    b) give as samples
    c) stock retail kits
    d) eat lunch

    A

55. Short and natural-looking is the best nail choice for a person who is a:
    a) computer operator
    b) telephone receptionist
    c) pianist
    d) stockbroker

    C

56. A good way to develop a steady clientele is to ask clients, before they leave the salon, to:
   a) buy retail
   b) make another appointment
   c) wash hands
   d) select polish

   B

57. The large, thick triangular muscle that covers the shoulder and lifts and turns the arm is called the:
   a) armature
   b) turner
   c) chloasma
   d) deltoid

   D

58. Because of the chemical hazards, a child present at your work station should be properly:
   a) supervised
   b) fed
   c) rested
   d) clothed

   A

59. The muscle which turns the hand outward so the palm faces upward is called the:
   a) terminator
   b) supinator
   c) pronator
   d) fibula

   B

60. Onyx is the technical term for:
   a) hair
   b) skin
   c) nails
   d) eyes

   C

61. Net income is the money you make less all your:
   a) expenses
   b) groceries
   c) clothes
   d) income

   A

62. Another name for hives is:
   a) hornets
   b) melanoma
   c) keratoma
   d) wheals

   D

63. Clear cells are found in the skin layer called:
   a) stratum corneum
   b) stratum lucidum
   c) melanin
   d) stratum mucosum

   B

64. A written description of services and prices is called the:
   a) job description
   b) promotions ad
   c) service list
   d) contract

   C

65. A light-colored, slightly raised mark on the skin formed after an injury or lesion of the skin has healed is called a/an:
   a) scar
   b) scratch
   c) abrasion
   d) callus

   A

66. The practice of offering only selected clients reduced prices should be:
   a) done discreetly
   b) a weekly ritual
   c) encouraged
   d) avoided

   D

67. Acrylic nails must be removed by soaking fingertips in:
   a) acetone
   b) baby oil
   c) cuticle remover
   d) alcohol

   A

68. Gel nails are applied by brushing the gel onto the:
   a) lunula
   b) cuticle
   c) entire nail
   d) primer

   C

69. No backup when you are gone is a disadvantage of working in:
   a) nails-only salon
   b) full-service salon
   c) your own salon
   d) selected areas

   B

70. The production of nail cells occurs in the nail:
    a) root
    b) bed
    c) matrix
    d) cuticle

    C

71. The clicking sound made by gently tapping the brush handle on an applied acrylic nail indicates the nails are:
    a) dry
    b) cracking
    c) new
    d) needing replacing

    A

72. Honesty is the best policy when dealing with a client's:
    a) polish
    b) objections
    c) nail file
    d) pedicure

    B

73. Income is the:
    a) money you make
    b) incoming client
    c) money you spend
    d) taxes due

    A

74. To speed the filing of long nails, first shorten them with a:
    a) nail buffer
    b) metal nail file
    c) fingernail clipper
    d) emery board

    C

75. The fingerbowl used during a manicure contains water and:
    a) alcohol
    b) antibacterial soap
    c) fungicide
    d) fumigants

    B

76. Metatarsal scissors is a massage movement which promotes:
    a) blood flow to neck
    b) blood flow to legs
    c) cutting ability
    d) flexibility

    D

77. An easy way for a nail technician to earn additional income is through:
    a) retail sales
    b) double-booking clients
    c) cleaning houses
    d) changing professions

    A

78. The slits or tracks in the nail bed at the sides of the nail on which the nail grows are called:
    a) slims
    b) rails
    c) grooves
    d) furrows

    C

79. An airbrush can be used with colored polish in nail art to create:
    a) shades and textures
    b) quick designs
    c) translucent applications
    d) gel nails base

    A

80. A temporary artificial nail service is a:
    a) mending job
    b) demonstration service
    c) tip with no overlay
    d) tip applied with water glue

    C

81. Rotation of elbow is a type of:
    a) chiropractic manipulation
    b) friction massage movement
    c) effleurage
    d) relaxer movement

    B

82. By spraying the client's nails with water, you can reduce the heat generated during:
    a) buffing
    b) acrylic removal
    c) polishing
    d) filing

    A

83. The half-moon shape at the base of the nail is called the:
    a) mantle
    b) matrix
    c) lunula
    d) groove

    C

84. An advantage of quats as a sanitation agent is their:
    a) stability
    b) weak solution
    c) odor
    d) bacteria

    A

85. This substance can be found in the stratum germinativum layer of the epidermis:
    a) elasticity
    b) mold
    c) herpes simplex
    d) melanin

    D

86. The service of trimming, shaping and polishing toenails, as well as performing foot massage, is called:
    a) podiatry
    b) manicuring
    c) pedicuring
    d) filing

    C

87. Circular movements in the palm is a massage technique known as:
    a) effleurage
    b) tapping
    c) friction massage
    d) joint relaxer movements

    A

88. Only half of the nail plate should be covered by a/an:
    a) glitter polish application
    b) artificial nail tip
    c) French Manicure polish
    d) buffer block

    B

89. Crack repair of an acrylic nail is performed using:
    a) silk wrap
    b) mending tissue
    c) acrylic
    d) clear polish

    C

90. The epidermis contains no:
    a) cells
    b) blood vessels
    c) nerves
    d) keratin

    B

91. Questions about a client's job are part of the:
    a) health information
    b) service record
    c) friendship process
    d) client profile

    D

92. The client's circulation is stimulated by:
    a) massage
    b) tip application
    c) buffing
    d) filing

    A

93. Tuberculocidal disinfectants are required to clean:
    a) toilet seats
    b) visible blood spills
    c) bathroom floor
    d) cuticle nippers

    B

94. The long, slender bones of the foot are called:
    a) metatarsals
    b) cartilage
    c) ligaments
    d) phalanges

    A

95. The excess skin beneath a toenail's free edge may be softened by using:
    a) alcohol
    b) silicone lotion
    c) cuticle solvent
    d) polish remover

    C

96. To avoid smearing polish, especially in a pedicure application, the top coat should be followed by:
    a) nail strengthener
    b) a second top coat
    c) hot blowing air
    d) instant nail dry

    D

97. Until you become accustomed to applying sculptured nails, support your work in progress by using two:
    a) brushes
    b) nail forms
    c) coats of top coat
    d) acrylic colors

    B

98. Always begin a manicure by working with the client's hand that is:
   a) not the favored one
   b) favored one
   c) in worse shape
   d) closest

   A

99. Skin that is red and sore is called:
   a) healthy
   b) infected
   c) inflamed
   d) circulated

   C

100. Gel nails stay the same color until:
   a) removed
   b) water cured
   c) buffed
   d) filed

   A